# HEALTHY DRINKS AND A HEALTHY LIFESTYLE FOR MEN

Healthy Food Nutrients & Biochemical Technology: including prayer and sports for all Christians as all people of Faith in Almighty God; and all people as created by God. [A.t.m.r]:

And how to seek God's spiritual blessings for a healthy lifestyle

By Caleb Chikomba Muzariri: B.Sc. Honours. Biochem.; M.Phil. Biochem.; M.Phil. Chem.Eng.

All rights reserved. This written and published book is copyright under the Berne convention and is published under the Copyright and Neighbouring Act. No part of this book may be reproduced, stored in a retrieval system or transmitted in any form or any means electronic, including photocopying, duplicating, recording without the permission in writing from the author, publisher and copyright holders. The unauthorized reproduction of this manuscript will constitute a copyright infringement and render the perpetrator liable under both civil and criminal law.

Caleb Chikomba Muzariri

Caleb's Genesis Publishers

19 Bromshill Drive, Cheetwood

Manchester, M7 4YT

United Kingdom

SCPF books: SCIENCE FOR CHRISTIANS & PEOPLE OF FAITH IN ALMIGHTY GOD: Book 1: by Caleb Chikomba Muzariri

ISBN 978-0-9926210-0-1   ©   Caleb's Genesis Publishers

**DEDICATION IN LOVE AND THANKS TO MY FAMILY:** I dedicate this book to my wife and all my children; who always make sure there is always clean cool water in the refrigerator for everyone to drink any time we need to drink water many times a day and all of the fruits you give me; except for only pomegranate that I fetch for myself!

**TO MY STUDENTS:** To all my former MBCHB second year medical students and my B.Sc. Honours Biochemistry students and M.Sc. Biotechnology students at University in Southern Africa from 1990 to 2004 & in the UK from 2004 onwards who always listened to my lectures or tutorials with interest each time I mentioned Jesus Christ Almighty God's power of creating the first molecules of life in the 'primordial soup' in forming the first living cell as He our living God created the universe, the earth, people and all living things (Genesis 1: 1 - 2).

**POTENTIAL READERS OF THIS BOOK:** This book is of interest to all men worldwide; and women worldwide to buy for their husbands; and all students of Medical Schools, Faith and Church Schools, Christian Universities, Bible Schools, all Colleges, Universities and Sports Clubs and Sportsmen; also Biochemists, Nutritionists, Physiotherapists and Health staff. The book describes fully nutrients in fruits & juices; and the technology of making some of the healthy drinks fresh in the home and how the nutrients can protect people against diseases by regular dietary intake at all age groups. The book also reminds people that God our creator is also the creator of everything that we eat and drink as much as he is also the creator of science capabilities for all mankind. The techniques of exercise and importance of physical exercise to a healthy lifestyle; and the physiological benefits of daily physical exercising to prevent disease are also described in this book. It is a handy reference for daily healthy nutrition and physical exercises; and a daily reminder of prayer to God.

**ACKNOWLEDGEMENTS:** I thank Professor Colin Webb of the University of Manchester Faculty of Engineering and Physical Sciences (formerly the world class UMIST) for being a good professional friend giving me insight into several possible PhD projects, one of which, time and funds allowing, would be nice for me to get going to complete, by the grace of God! I also thank Archbishop Professor Ezekiel H. Guti of the FIFMI Church for his humble teachings on how to be a humble man of God, to put trust and to believe in our Lord Jesus Christ as our living God whom we should seek first every day for guidance before doing any other personal tasks (James 4: 10; Matthew 18: 4; Mark 16: 16-18; Romans 10: 9-11). I also thank my local Pastor and Provincial Overseer, Reverend Thadaeus Mike (the spiritual son of Professor Guti) for prayers to our living God, Jesus Christ, who provides and enables us everything good in our lives.

**SPECIAL TRIBUTE:** In special tribute to my beloved parents Baba Joel T. Muzariri and Mai Rebecca Muzariri (both then being devoted leading Evangelists of the Methodist Church) who taught me as a child how to pray to our Lord Jesus Christ (Proverbs 22: 6) and how to be a scientist who believes in God (Daniel 1: 3 – 20; Daniel 3: 25 – 30).

**TO ALL MEN OF GOD:** This book will also enable all husbands to advise their loving wives on healthy drinks and foods that give good and nutritional protection from long term diseases such as cancers and preventing blood pressures in the long term. God created Adam and Eve for He so loved man and woman to always love each other and to enjoy one another and that plan for all mankind by Almighty God will never change (Genesis 2: 22 – 25).

*"And they were all filled with the Holy Spirit and began to speak with other tongues, as the spirit gave them utterance"* (Acts 2: 4).

| CONTENTS | |
|---|---|
| COPYRIGHT STATEMENT | 1 |
| DEDICATION | 2 |
| AKNOWLEDGEMENTS | 3 |
| SPECIAL TRIBUTE | 3 |
| CHAPTER ONE: The importance of clean drinking water since Biblical Genesis. Health benefits of drinking fresh natural water. Drinking plenty of water for good health. | 7 |
| Commercially purified water. The technology of filtration and purifying your own domestic water. | |
| CHAPTER TWO: Drinking water with other healthy supplements. Taking vitamin C with plenty water. Multivitamin daily with plenty water. | 16 |
| Health benefits of vitamin C; protection against cancer, heart diseases, against diabetes. Health benefits of multivitamins supplement; health boost. | |
| CHAPTER THREE: Healthy sugar-free drinks to prevent diabetes. | 20 |
| Natural sugar-free drinks; water, green tea, black tea; healthy nutrients in green tea, black tea; health benefits of sugar-free drinks. | |
| CHAPTER FOUR: Healthy natural power drinks for athletes, footballers and other sportsmen. | 22 |
| The natural sportsman and normal diet. The natural sportsman taking no alcohol, no smoking, no toxic substances. | |
| CHAPTER FIVE: Drinking soya milk with honey or as plain milk. Healthy nutrients in soya milk; benefits. | 28 |
| Industrial production of soya milk. Honey formation from healthy natural nectar by bees; health benefits from honey. How to farm your own honey bees. | |

| CONTENTS | |
|---|---|
| CHAPTER SIX: Healthy red coloured and blue coloured fruit juices and mixtures. | 34 |
| Pomegranate, cranberry, tomato, red grapes, red guava, strawberry, prune (dried plum) juices; healthy nutrients in the juices; health benefits and protection against diseases and against aging. | |
| CHAPTER SEVEN: Mixed tropical and other fruits juices. Typical mixture of banana, mango, orange, lemon, pineapple, melon, apple, peach, tomato and pomegranate. | 43 |
| Healthy nutrients in the fruits juice; health benefits and protection against diseases and against aging.<br>The technology of producing your own fresh fruit juice. | |
| CHAPTER EIGHT: Healthy hot beverages | 56 |
| Hot cocoa; hot chocolates; diet chocolates; healthy nutrients; health benefits and protection against disease; vitality, longetivity and healthy life benefits. | |
| CHAPTER NINE: Healthy hot soups with no salt added | 62 |
| Mushroom soup & health benefits; chicken soup; broccoli soup; tomato soup; healthy nutrients. | |
| CHAPTER TEN: Other citrus fruits | 68 |
| Avocado, black mulberries, lemon fruit juice & honey anti-flu tonic; the need to always pray to Almighty God our living Lord Jesus Christ who gives us all the healthy fruits benefits . | |
| CHAPTER ELEVEN: Making healthy non-alcoholic drinks from sorghum and millet. | 73 |
| Brewing the non-alcoholic beverages; healthy nutrients in sorghum and millets. The potential technology improvements. | |

| CONTENTS | |
|---|---|
| CHAPTER TWELVE: Making healthy fermented fruit and milk products: yogurts. | 80 |
| Method 1: Yogurt making technology; Method 2: Yogurt making: lactose-free yogurt making technology; health benefits of yogurts and protection against diseases. | |
| CHAPTER THIRTEEN: Healthy endurance training and maximum preparation to be top world class athlete or sportsman. | 84 |
| Some good hints and training comments from a former world class athlete. The techniques of top sprinting. | |
| CHAPTER FOURTEEN: How to exercise and keep fit as a man, daily. The healthy lifestyle of tithing at your local church to thank God for good health and all healthy benefits. | 89 |
| Physical exercises; physiological and biochemical benefits of exercising; anti-aging and diseases prevention; personal enjoyment satisfaction and good health. | |
| DAILY INSPIRATION: The importance of prayer to our living God Jesus Christ and thanking God's blessings for a healthy lifestyle. | 96 |
| | |
| INDEX | 101 |

# CHAPTER ONE

## THE IMPORTANCE OF CLEAN DRINKING WATER SINCE BIBLICAL GENESIS

1. BAPTISM WATER AND THE HOLY SPIRIT FOR THE BLESSED CHRISTIAN WHO BELIEVES IN OUR LORD JESUS CHRIST AND TAKES HIM TO BE OUR SAVIOUR FROM SINS: As a believer in our Lord Jesus Christ, I also believe that He our Living God enables me to interpret the principles, applications and practices of modern science more accurately and more effectively. In this regard the Baptism water becomes a very healthy drink to the new born again Christian as it cleanses the inner soul from sins and leaves the heart clean, filled with His love and the Holy Spirit. A good Christian not only becomes redeemed from sin but from many diseases; and the Christian's body becomes very much rejuvenated with good physical health as well as spiritual health (Acts 2: 3 - 4). The Holy Spirit renews our body by renewing also our body cells by faith, replacing the old diseased cells with new healthy ones that are freed from the disease of sin. Therefore drinking the Baptism water either through your skin as you are immersed in it or as you swallow a bit of it through the mouth during the Baptism immersion, is therefore partaking in a very healthy drink that also blesses you with the Holy Spirit on that day of Baptism (John 1: 25). Our Lord Jesus Christ taught by example by Himself being baptized in water (Matthew 3: 16-17). The added benefit after taking the Baptism water is the promise of everlasting life from our Heavenly Father our JEHOVAH, Mighty God who so loved us that He gave to us His only begotten Son Lord Jesus Christ to die for the remission of our sins on the cross as Thomas and other

disciples touched Him for us to strengthen our faith (Luke 24:39-40). After water Baptism, when the Holy Spirit enters into your lifestyle, the Holy Spirit encourages you the new man of integrity to walk away from sins. The Holy Spirit anoints you and blesses you to prosper, keeping you away from drinking unhealthy drinks such as beer, intoxicating distilled liquors and intoxicating wines or toxic drugs. A newly born again believer of Lord Jesus Christ is blessed by the Holy Spirit to live a healthy lifestyle that is always sober, comforting and very pleasing to their wives as this same Holy Spirit in the men makes the wives feel safe and loved in their sober husband's hands.

2. REAL NATURAL CLEAN WATER OR PURE SPRING WATER IS THE BEST AND CHEAPEST DRINK FOR GOOD HEALTH AS WE RECEIVE IT FREE FROM ALMIGHTY GOD'S RAIN:
And let us all thank God for the water whether you are Christian or not because at one time the Prophet Elijah actually asked God to stop the rain for 3 years and there was such great suffering without it; that Elijah was forced to pray hard again to ask God to bring it back! (James 5: 17-18). There was so much acute suffering without water during Elijah's 3 years of no rain. People must have suffered poor health, severe malnutrition, dehydrations, severe blood circulatory problems, besides the obvious hunger and thirst without the rain water (1Kings 17: 1-24, 1Kings 18: 41-45). Elijah was a very faithful man as He obeyed God's instructions in his prayers for the rain and water; that Almighty God took him to heaven alive
(2 Kings 2: 11-15). At another time our Almighty God was so angry with the recalcitrant sinners that He warned Noah and his family to build quickly an Ark before God

flooded the whole earth with the rain water (Genesis 6, 7 and 8); but our living God so loves us that He has assured us that no more such drastic punishment will happen to us all those who receive Jesus Christ as our Saviour who died for the remission of our sins. We are now therefore blessed with abundant healthy water to drink from the rain water, whilst our sins are forgiven when we accept Jesus Christ as our only Saviour. We can now drink as much water as we like to keep ourselves very healthy. Water keeps us very healthy in many ways when we drink it properly. After almost being dumped for dead by his mother Hagar, Ishmael was later saved by his mother giving him water to drink from a well God had just shown her as she prayed faithfully (Genesis 21: 15-21). Because of the importance of good clean water to drink and to survive, there was almost a war between Abraham and Abimelech, which Abraham being a man of God peacefully resolved (Genesis 21: 25 – 33). The Biblical romance between Isaac and Rebecca took place at a clean drinking water well where Rebecca had gone to fetch water *pa tsime* (Genesis 24). At another clean drinking water well; *pa tsime ra* Jacob (at Jacob's well), our Lord Jesus Christ sat tired and thirsty and said to the Samaria woman: "Give me to drink." (John 4: 7).

3. HEALTH BENEFITS OF DRINKING PLENTY OF CLEAN FRESH WATER REGULARLY AND A HEALTHY LIFESTYLE FOR MEN:

Really fresh and clean water from rain or natural springs is simply the pure liquid $H_2O$. Being the pure clean liquid that it is, when we drink it, we are also adding something clean and pure into our body system through of course the stomach and digestive tract. Water is easily absorbed throughout our digestive tract carrying with it to our blood stream, all the digested food molecules such as the healthy amino acids, peptides and short chain proteins, vitamins, fatty acids, simple sugars and complex carbohydrates, minerals, antioxidants and biological salts that our bodies need for normal function to activate enzymes of overall healthy body metabolic activities. The pancreas produces the sugar regulating insulin hormone more efficiently when we drink plenty of fresh clean water without overloading our bodies with other things in the water. Therefore simply drinking pure clean water before and after meals keeps us safe from 'overeating' diseases such as diabetes and obesity because with water drinking only, we are not poisoning our bodies with anything else. Water is also very good for clearing off a build-up of body toxins through enhanced kidney filtration and removal of such toxins into urine that we pass out of our bodies in large amounts after drinking plenty of water. For example if one is feeling uncomfortable and suspecting poisoning causing high blood pressure problems; the first wise self-medication is to drink plenty of water. Drinking plenty of water increases the chances of getting rid of the high blood pressure (bps) causing toxins and can well prevent the need for prescribed medications for bps control. For men such self-medication of bps with drinking plenty of water is very important because men's libido can be quickly ruined by premature medication with prescribed bps control medications and once the men's libido goes, it is not only the man that worries and suffer but also the man's wife also worries for losing the sexual satisfaction from her husband because of premature medication of the bps controlling prescribed drugs which then would be required to be taken for life! instead of the bps being managed by self-medication control by simply drinking plenty of water to control the bps. The healthy man can always feel extremely good, strong and very active after he administers to himself with very large amounts of clean filtered water and bottled water to keep himself feeling healthy and bps-free not only for his own good but for the good also of the wife! God also wants all men to be wise so as to satisfy their wives by keeping a healthy physically and spiritually because God does not want men to deprive their wives sexually (1 Corinthians 7: 1 - 7). Therefore the first line of self-defence for any man against bps diseases, diabetes, obesity and loss of libido is to be very faithful to self-prescribing oneself daily, more than 2 litres of clean water to drink per day so as to drive through the body, food molecules coming from also healthy foods and to ensure that the kidneys are efficiently removing most of the toxins into the large volume of water urine waste. Drinking large volumes of clean water daily is also a very good way of keeping the kidneys healthy as they are carrying out their most natural function of filtering from the body, plenty of water and the toxins.

4. USE OF COMMERCIALLY PURIFIED WATER AND CLEAN WATER DURING SPORTS AND ATHLETICS; OR DURING OTHER ACTIVITIES BY MAN:

Our bodies lose a lot of water through sweating the moment we are subjected to any intense form of exercise. In warm to hot weather, there is a higher rate of loss of water by sweating and perspiring leading to large volumes of water going out from our bodies. Man therefore needs to quickly replace that water being lost through sweat during exercises of any kind. The exercising individual needs to regularly drink purified, good standard quality tested commercially supplied clean water at the chosen intervals so as to rehydrate the body quickly. Rehydration is very important because, if on the other hand, excessive dehydration is let to occur; the body will build up toxins as the kidneys are deprived of adequate water to carry away the salts and other toxins from the body. Such dehydration can then cause the individual to suffer possible organ and body tissues poisoning causing poor health to the individual. Water is the best rehydrating agent for everyone sensible during exercises. It is therefore important to set up a self-reliant domestic clean water supply so as avoid the costs of buying every time commercial bottled water, especially when the keen sportsmen will also want to produce own clean fruit juices and other beverages from guaranteed bacteria-free and pollutants-free clean water. Section 4.1 therefore deals with the technology of setting up a clean water filtration and purification system in your own home.

**4.1** DOMESTIC WATER TREATMENT TECHNOLOGY: THE USE OF PRE-HOUSE WATER FILTRATION SYSTEMS FOR WHOLE HOUSE AND DRINKING WATER MICROFILTRATION SYSTEMS IN THE KITCHEN:

> It is important to ensure that water coming from the general public supply works is sufficiently clean and hygienic and safe for own personal needs especially as we must drink for good health minimum of 2 litres of water per day. If there is any doubt about cleanliness and health safety of the general house water supply; it is advised to fit your own independent standard house water filtration system to the pipe that comes to the whole house.

**4.2** FITTING INTO PLACE THE STANDARD WHOLE HOUSE WATER FILTRATION SYSTEM:

The largest Standard Whole House Water Filtration System is designed for household of more than 5 people and has the capacity to filter 600 000 litres per year before you change the filtration cartridge. It is designed to be fitted by any DIY plumber where the water pipe enters the house. This has a 5 micron filter that removes sediment or sludge. It is fitted with a carbon block cartridge that filters off 99.9% of chlorine from your public supplied water; including removing pesticides, herbicides, phenols and volatile organic carbons. It is robust and effective and should not cost too much to buy and install including plumbing charges. Since this system initially cleans the incoming house water, to ensure guaranteed healthy drinking water, it is important to fit into the kitchen, a Drinking Water Filtration system of your own choice.

## 4.3 FITTING THE DOMESTIC DRINKING WATER FILTRATION SYSTEM:

This system should not also cost too much to buy and install, unless you decide to scale up your filtration for purposes beyond domestic, which then becomes more expensive. There are many types of Drinking Water Filtration Systems in the market depending on your own personal preferences. Most drinking water filtration systems are fitted by your DIY plumber under the kitchen sink; others are fitted within the top cupboards of your kitchen. One of the most interesting one is the model drinking water filtration system that operates with electronic touch buttons to select whether you want cold water or ordinary water or warm water and also the quantity of water to dispense out. This model is fitted on top of your kitchen cupboard if you prefer the electronics of it. But there are also many other similar varieties in the market; choose carefully according to long term maintenance costs.

> The under the sink varieties are also many in the market. One interesting type has a 5 micron filter pad that has high performance with a bacterio-static medium. This removes chlorine, lead, arsenic and mercury from water. This system also has a silver-impregnated carbon that protects the filtration media from back contamination bacteria. Granular activated carbon protects drinking water from chemical compounds. In addition there is

riolyte that makes drinking water taste palatable. To confirm that the extruded carbon filter cartridge is actually solid chemical adsorption matrix that actually works, US Patent 5164085A describes the Cartridge as: consisting of 3 layers of adsorption materials: i. The 10 microns pore size outer pre-filtration layer; ii. The 5 microns pore size central adsorption layer; iii. The inner 0.9 microns filter layer of ceramic impregnated with silver to trap pathogenic microorganisms such as *Escherica Coli, Typhoid, Cholera* and *Cryptosporidium* and heavy metals; other chemicals such as chlorine and organic compounds.

## 4.4 THE COMMERCIAL UNDER THE SINK WATER FILTRATION AND PURIFICATION SYSTEMS:

A typical commercial under the sink water filtration and purification system can produce more than 2000 litres per day of bacteria-free, microbial-free and toxic metals-free high quality water. Such a system is very good for those countries where public water health and safety presents challenging problems; especially some developing countries where water resources management is riddled with corrupt officials who do not do their job properly; forcing communities to team up together to supply each other with safe clean water.

A basic under the sink commercial reverse osmosis filtration system can be found from the market; designed to fit under the sink without need for a tank or a pump. It carries out reverse osmosis filtration whilst allowing the tap to operate at a reasonable flow rate of over 2000 litres of high quality water per day; being suitable for the domestic kitchen. The reverse osmosis system is very robust; removing 99.9% of each of the following contaminants encountered by communities experiencing dirty water problems: removes 99.9% bacteria, protozoa, amoeba,

Sodium, Calcium, Magnesium, Aluminium, Copper, Nickel, Chlorine, Lead, Cadmium, Silver and Bicarbonates, Borates. If it is operating daily at maximum capacity; only one cartridge filter needs to be changed after 6 months. Post filtration testing of water quality can be done routinely to confirm high standard pure water quality; by ordering suitable water testing kits. A good quality cartridge filter can be available made from an extruded activated carbon block combined with natural cocoanut shell carbon to ensure enhanced drinking water health safety standard.

Just for comparison, a typical small scale industrial system is scaled up to produce nearly 5000 litres per day and it requires a tank.

Ref.US:Patent:5164085A:WaterFilterCartridge; dwi.defra.gov.uk/consumer/advice:2010;www.uk-water-filters.co.uk;www.eastmidlandswater.com; www.virginpure.com; www.eaucoolers.co.uk/waterfilters; www.faireyfiltersdirect.com; www.nef.org; www.healthy-house.co.uk

# CHAPTER TWO
## DRINKING WATER TOGETHER WITH OTHER HEALTHY NUTRIENT SUPPLEMENTS

1. TAKING WATER WITH VITAMIN SUPPLEMENTS AND NUTRIENTS

The general well-being, vitality and happiness of every man is both important to the man himself, his wife and his children. Wives like strong, energetic and adventurous husbands in the bedroom and not lethargic, weak and clueless men in the holy matrimony. The outward going vibrant witty brain and robust body build needs vitamin supplements to keep the men healthy and alert to the demands and challenges of modern day life. Generally the food we eat, even though it may be very nutritious and healthy may still not be enough for a healthy outgoing man especially also that kind of man who works very hard for every day of the week. To keep the man in top form, it is therefore wise for the man to select his own choice of vitamin supplements that suit his own lifestyle and daily activities. The story of Abraham and Sarah in the Bible is very illustrative of how men must always be very prepared to satisfy their wives even at advanced age of 100 years old! (Genesis 17: 17). Abraham pleased both his wife Sarah and God Himself by being strong and faithful enough to perform on Sarah as God had pre-destined him to do ( Genesis 17: 1 -17). Abraham rejuvenated Sarah by making her conceive at the age of over 90 years and Sarah was the most pleased woman to give birth to her son Isaac at that very late age (Genesis 18: 10 -15). She actually laughed when God initially told her she was going to have a child at that age but Abraham remained faithful and kept himself strong to perform for the promise (Genesis 18 10 -15). Abraham was a clever man who kept himself very strong and healthy for his wife Sarah's needs and not his own needs alone. Indeed Abraham must have used some good source of vitamin supplements, especially from his favoured butter, milk and other good sources, to keep his vitality going strong (Genesis 18: 8). Sarah was also a very clever woman who highly respected her husband lifting up his dignity by calling him Lord and feeding him well making sure he was drinking healthy drinks only; not beer or other intoxicating things. Abraham was a sober man of God and very faithful to God and faithful to his wife Sarah who so loved him that she gave him another woman Hagar to have a child with. There is no fear in true love (1 John 4: 18 - 19).

When taking daily vitamin supplements, an individual may either choose to take either only one vitamin supplement such as one vitamin C tablet per day or a tablet of several vitamins called the multivitamin tablet, also normally one tablet per day; each vitamin tablet being taken with adequate daily intake of water not less than 2 litres per day.

2. THE HEALTH BENEFITS OF TAKING DAILY ONE TABLET OF VITAMIN C SUPPLEMENT WITH ADEQUATE DAILY WATER INTAKE:

Vitamin C is biochemically known by ourselves Biochemists as Ascorbic acid and known to be one of the most powerful vitamins for a man's healthy lifestyle. Men need to take in sufficient or even surplus daily amount of the vitamin C against many forms of cancer, such as against bowl cancer, organ cancers and prostate cancer from a very young age of their manhood, through middle age and old age; throughout their lives. It is a potentially very protective vitamin because it is well known for its very potent anti-oxidant properties to destroy toxic radicals from the body that, without vitamin C oxidation effect, such toxic radicals could cause cancers to the individual. Naturally, vitamin C is found in almost all the fresh fruits, vegetables and tomatoes that we eat. But daily fruit and salad vegetable consumption alone does not give enough of the protective amounts of vitamin C required for a man's protection against cancers and therefore to be on the safe side, all men must always take vitamin C in with enough daily water, the daily supplementary tablet of vitamin C; which is very safe of course because it is basically a sweet and fruity vitamin; so why not enjoy it for own maximum health benefits?

Adam and Eve originally were allowed by God to live in the abundantly fruity Garden of Eden (Genesis 1 - 13) so as to enjoy maximum health benefits with all the rich vitamin C resource they could get from all the fruits in the garden. But Satan deceived Eve to disobey God by making her eat that special fruit which probably God was reserving for them for a special celebration with Him and them as indeed God later told them they had eaten the fruit from the tree of life that should give eternal life (Genesis 3: 21 – 22); and she sinfully passed on the special stolen fruit to her husband Adam. Both man and wife got the curse of generations for all mankind because they both got tempted for the special vitamin C in that special fruit of God! After eating that forbidden fruit, we are told by the Bible that suddenly the pair discovered that they were naked and tried to hide from God! (Genesis 1: 1 - 13). What a hopeless situation our two parents found themselves in; but we are required by God to respect them for they remain our parents up to now and forever! For it is written children honour your parents (Colossians 3:10; Ephesians 6: 1 - 3). Indeed we must all honour them so that our own days are multiplied to eternal life; through the Holy Spirit blessings as per promise by God to Abraham (1 John 2: 24 – 25) and our redemption by our LORD Jesus Christ (Matthew 26: 28).

3. THE HEALTH BENEFITS OF TAKING IN ONE DAILY SUPPLEMENT OF A FULL MULTIVITAMIN TABLET WITH ADEQUATE DAILY WATER INTAKE:

The best multivitamin tablet must always contain the following composition of vitamins: Vitamin A, Vitamin D,

Vitamin E, Vitamin K, Vitamin C, Vitamin B1 (Thiamine), Vitamin B2 (Riboflavin), Niacin, Vitamin B6, Folic acid, Vitamin B12, Biotin, Pantothenic acid, Calcium, Magnesium, Iron, Manganese, Selenium, Chromium, Iodine, Coenzyme Q10. In addition to these, some probiotic supplements contain friendly intestinal bacteria that carry out health enhancing intestinal fermentations to enhance the overall vitality of a highly active man daily.

Vitamin A is beta carotene which is naturally abundant in carrots and is good for a healthy eye sight. It is also called retinol and is fat soluble. It is an antioxidant and has anti-cancer metabolic activity. The health benefits of vitamin D, E, K, C, B1, B2, B6, B12 and the rest of the other vitamins and minerals are fully described in Chapter 7 as nutrients present in fresh fruits. Iodine is important as a supplement to prevent the clinical condition called goitre, abnormal growth, mental and physical retardation and other body metabolic problems. Iodine controls the thyroid gland which produces thyroid hormones. Thyroid hormones regulate many metabolic activities of body cells, tissues and organs. Pregnant women need daily adequate iodine amounts to ensure normal healthy baby development and to prevent cretinism.

REFERENCE: S. Harakech, A.J. Jariwalla and L. Pauling (1990). Showing Vitamin C as a potent suppressor of HIV activation: Proceedings of National Acad. Sc. USA: 87(18) 7245 – 7259 (September 1990).

www.organicfacts.net/healthbenefitsofminerals.May 2013

# CHAPTER THREE

## HEALTHY SUGAR FREE DRINKS TO PREVENT DIABETES

### NATURAL SUGAR FREE DRINKS AVAILABLE

**Water** is the best known sugar free drink to get used to. Different sources of clean bottled water are now available in supermarkets in almost all countries of the world.

Other recommended natural sugar free drinks include black tea, green tea and black coffee.

Carbonated beverages are not healthy for proper prevention of diabetes because they contain too much added sweetener that has long term side effects on health.

**Green tea** is made from unfermented leaves which are rich in the natural antioxidants.

Green tea benefits to health are as follows: it is rich in catechin polyphenols antioxidants called epigallocatechin gallate which destroy cancer cells without damage to the healthy tissue cells. Green tea also lowers cholesterol levels and prevents blood platelets from clotting thereby protecting the cardiovascular circulatory system from defective blood flow and bps. Green tea also prevents dental decay by destroying plaque forming bacteria. It is also known to prevent diabetes and reducing incidence of dementia. Green tea also prevents aesophagus cancer and has a wide antiviral action against influenza and cancers.

Green tea also promotes increased fat metabolism resulting in the higher burning rate of body fats, causing overall weight loss. The effect of theannine, an amino acid found in green tea is known to be good as a tranquilizer and relaxing agent that prevents depression.

Researchers have recently shown that green tea prevents the growth of prostate cancer cells, lung cancer cells, skin cancer, pancreatic cancer and stomach cancer.

It is however **warned** not to take green tea during chemotherapy and after taking blood clotting medications and to consult your doctor before using green tea.

**Black tea** has similar health benefits to green tea. Black tea contains more tannins that boost the immune system against many diseases such as influenza, dysentery and hepatitis.

Above all these drinks and natural remedies, all men who believe that Jesus Christ is our only Saviour and our only living God, should always remember to pray; so as to hand over all your troubles to Almighty God for the healing of your troubles or disease by the Holy Spirit of our Lord Jesus who said 'by His Stripes at the Cross and by His heavenly powers and grace you are healed in the name of Jesus Christ'; or pray to simply thank God for the excellent health He is giving you if you have no troubles.

REFERENCE: Eric W.C. Chan, Eu Ying Soh, Pei Pei Tie and Yon Peng Law: Antooxidant and antibacterial properties of green, black and herbal teas of *Camellia sinensis*. Pharmacology Research 2011 October – December 3 (4): 266 – 271.

www.umm.edu. University of Maryland Medical Centre: May 2013

# CHAPTER FOUR

## HEALTHY POWER DRINKS FOR ATHLETES, FOOTBALLERS AND OTHER SPORTSMEN

1. THE NATURAL SPORTSMAN AND NORMAL DIET: *Is it really necessary for athletes and other sportsmen to medicate themselves with all sorts of chemicals and substances so as to be champions*? I begin here with my own personal story as a very successful athlete winning several medals at my College during my school days. My friend and I belonged to the same school House of Sports at our then Boarding school. By an interesting coincidence that friend of mine happened to be one of the two best 100 meters and 200 meters athletes also in the whole College outside our own Sports House that we both represented. Belonging to the same House club as such, made us so intensely competitive of each other about who would beat the other if we did not avoid each other in a race tournament. Personally I decided to go secretly for intense field sprinting practices and doing the gym exercises secretly, especially lifting weights so as to build my muscles in both legs and arms. I did not know that my friend was also secretly intensely training similarly also. For a long time the two of us always avoided racing each, but would plot opposing teams by running at separate events and of course only the relays put us together; which our team always won convincingly thanks to the two of us being in the same relay team. Even our coach was kind of collaborator in making sure we did not race each out within the same team. The crunch race between my friend and I came when a new coach took over to prepare the whole boarding school team for National Athletic finals of all top athletes from many Schools and

Colleges in that country. One final preparation arrived and the coach curiously wanted to know the proper sprint record of the school between my friend and I on the 100 meters. So for the first time the two of us were finally forced to race 100 meters sprint against dear friend. This event was well attended by the whole school who also wanted to know who was really the champion between my friend and I. Timing clocks and time recorders were properly set up in place by the coach for this race because he wanted to see the proper school record for 100 meters sprint between my friend and I. In this very special event we were also joined in the competition by 3 other very strong stars from other competing groups, so it was not guaranteed that only my friend or I would be champion of the race. Finally the race starter lined us up and coolly waited before blowing the race starter gun: all of us 6 strong sprinters surged with POWER FORWARD FOR THE WIN. The result was amazing to the time recorders. My friend and I not only tied deadlock at the school championship new record; my friend and I had set a new school record tied together. The judges checked out our then new 100 meter record with the national SENIOR record and were amazed that we had also set a new national record; on further checks, by the judges, the judges said we had actually 'unofficially' set the new world record, 9.94s, of that year! This result was not taken seriously by both the judges and my friend and I for several reasons. Firstly some judges mumbled that we had been wind assisted to make the 'unofficial' world record. Up to now I have never really understood the term wind assisted for champion athletes! The second reason to ignore my friend and I 'unofficial' world record was the hard fact that our school was not registered for international professional athletics championships and so even our school recording judges were being questioned as to their recording accuracy. Thirdly our coach also knew that even if we had 'unofficially' clocked a new world record for the 100 meters, neither me nor my friend was ever going to get any sponsorship because the country for which we did it was under United Nations sanctions due to serious political offences by the then political leaders of that country.

*Back to the point in question: is it really necessary for athletes to medicate themselves with all sorts of chemicals and substances so as to be champions?* From the above described 'unofficial' new world record on 100 meters then set by my friend and I, I say that my answer <u>is strictly no</u> to any so called performance enhancing substances but yes to natural muscle strengthening and building through tough training endurance and the strong physical gym training. And yes also to hard work practice on the actual track so as to be real champions! As my friend and I almost became world champions if we were in the right country at the right time! My personal diet at that Boarding school frequently started with porridge with milk in the morning for breakfast; Maize meal and vegetables at lunch time; Rice and any meat, beef or chicken or fish for supper. My snack was brown sugar in 500ml of bottled water, that was, famously nicknamed 'koro' drink by all at the Boarding school; the 'koro' drink taken together with a bread sandwich of peanut butter; famously called 'dovi' at the boarding school those days. So with that very basic diet I was that very near the real world 100 metre championship record through physical training of muscles and not by taking any chemicals! It is my strong opinion that all good athletics champions should be as similarly natural as much as possible to be real natural athletes champions, of course using the modern natural diet that has also vastly improved with plenty of new good food recipes and healthy drinking products to naturally build the athlete's body. I must also add here that personally I grew up at my father's farm where I always had abundant fruits with plenty of vitamins. My father also used to keep plenty of bees hives on the farm and I always ate plenty of honey. This makes me faithful to the healthy vitamin rich natural fresh fruits drinks and honey to be part of a good sportsman's diet and training kit; not chemical substances of sorts.

2. THE NATURAL STRONG SPORTSMAN TAKING NO ALCOHOL, NO SMOKING AND NO DRUGS, NO CORRUPT TOXIC ENHANCERS:

For a good start, a good athlete must firstly be very self-disciplined to a clean, sober and healthy lifestyle of no to alcohol, no to tobacco smoking and no to drugs and no to any artificial enhancing substances. Such a clean, sober athlete has the greatest chance of one day making it to the greatest of all world stages, the Olympics, firstly without being shamed by people, but as a real people's hero; and secondly, with greater chances of being blessed by our living God Jesus Christ who happens to be the first friend and companion of the good people of the earth who do no sin or indulge in corrupt practices of all sorts. So with God's blessings, such a clean athlete is already a winner, for there is an adept scripture quote that says: "God gives us according to His riches in the glory of our Lord Jesus Christ." Therefore a clean and completely sober lifestyle is the only guaranteed road to a great athlete and sportsman of great honour and praise by people; with possible heavenly blessings and benefits from our almighty God. When I clocked the 'unofficial' 100 metre world records; I thank God that at that youthful time, indeed I too was a clean, sober young man of only about 18 years old and so I can afford to also write about it and laugh about it here in this book! Because I still feel good about it even today, many years later! I am not saying I was a spruce perfect young man all the time, but I am simply saying at that particular time and event I was absolutely clean and sober and I feel good and free for that! But if I had that time knowingly tainted myself with bad substances, I do not think and see how the guilt of such an unclean practice would even allow me to write this chapter in this book. This remark I have just made here is advice and warning to all the young athletes and sportsmen to keep sober and clean, even for the distant future's clean record sake; whereby you will want to look back many years later and still feel fresh good that it was well worth it to keep clean and sober as you made your own world records; because you might want to also write about them as I am doing right now and feel proud about it! Therefore to all young athletes and all aspiring world champions of tomorrow; just now keep clean, sober and enjoy a healthy lifestyle for even tomorrow's sake and you will be proud of your 'record' achievement years later.  I am not writing my whole biography but just stating a specific point of good youthful discipline; which also thank God, I attribute to my own strong Christian parents who did not allow me to indulge into anything stupid as a young man then. There you kids out there, listen to and obey your parents because years later, you will like that record of a healthy young lifestyle; and do yourself a favour to read the Bible because that is also definitely God's guaranteed healthy lifestyle for all young people; and you parents out there read Proverbs 22:6 in the Holy Bible and find out what I mean. Therefore as far as possible the best power drink of a good, clean athlete and sportsman is taking in the Holy Spirit from almighty God, drinking God created clean natural fruits juices, water and the natural vitamins and natural nutrients (Genesis 43:11); so as to keep a clean, sober and healthy lifestyle; and practising hard on the track and working out hard in the gym. A good sportsman or simply every active man should be enterprising; buy yourself a fruit juice making machine and make yourself and your family real fresh fruit juice of your choice daily from farm fruits or wholesale fruits. Buy yourself also a water filter system to make yourself clean water daily so as to store adequate cold water in the refrigerator. Sweeten your fresh fruit juice only with natural honey if it is necessary to sweeten the fruit juice or filtered water. That way you are on your way to a healthy financial independence on natural fresh fruit juices and clean filtered water; and a healthy life style for you and family. In the Holy Bible we read about Esau being one of those athletes who enjoyed natural nutrients to keep himself fit; but this time Esau over did by selling his birthright for Jacob's 'red pottage of lentils' (Genesis 25: 30 – 34).

OTHER BIBLE READINGS: Genesis 43: 34; Genesis 49: 12; Psalm 103, Psalm 104, Psalm 113 and Psalm 150.

# CHAPTER FIVE

## DRINKING SOYA MILK WITH HONEY OR AS PLAIN MILK

1. ### THE NATURAL NUTRIENTS MOLECULAR COMPOSITION OF SOYA MILK THAT MAKES IT A HEALTHY DRINK:

Table 1.1: Soya milk contains the following:

| NUTRIENT | AMOUNT IN 100ML |
|---|---|
| PROTEIN | 3.4g |
| SUGARS | 0.1g |
| UNSATURATED FAT | 1.6g |
| SATURATED FATS | 0.3g |
| MONO-UNSATURATES | 0.4g |
| POLYUNSATURATES | 1.2g |
| FIBRE | 0.6g |
| SODIUM | TRACE |
| RECOMMENDED VITAMIN/MINERALS DAILY | |
| VITAMIN D | 0.8mcg |
| RIBOFLAVIN | 0.2mcg |
| VITAMIN B12 | 0.4mcg |
| CALCIUM | 120mg |

### 1.1 THE HEALTH BENEFITS OF DRINKING SOYA MILK:

Soya milk is well known to have 6 major health benefits: namely improved body lipids profile; strengthening blood vessels; promoting weight loss; preventing prostate cancer; preventing post-menopausal syndrome and preventing osteoporosis.

Improvement of the body lipids profile arises from the special nutrient lipids that originate from the soya bean. The soya milk contains rich source of only unsaturated fatty acids and has no cholesterol, unlike cow milk which has saturated fats and cholesterol. Cholesterol is major cause of cardiovascular diseases and bps. Drinking soya milk daily is known to actually reduce cholesterol levels and to improve overall health and well-being of people. Recently on the other hand, unfortunately soya milk high levels of the 6 omega unsaturated has been suspected to causing other adverse effects such as diabetes and therefore it is now advised to take soya not in excess, preferably with an alternative source of the good 3 Omega unsaturated fats. This adverse effect of soya milk's 6 Omega is an expected fact of life that not even one of the many other natural drink extracts are totally free from their own defects and shortcomings and therefore it will always remain grandmother's old advice that too much of anything is no good! And therefore we must always be careful to balance all our fruit drinks or cereal extracts drinks to prevent unexpected health pitfalls from one hostile substance or other within our favourite natural drinks! Therefore for example despite the 6 Omega problem, soya milk remains important to lower bps and is a must for those allergic to cow milk; and of course it is a new challenge for Biochemists and other scientists to find ways to produce 6 Omega-free new soya milk soon, and that means new varieties of soya beans that are 6 Omega-free!

The health benefit of strengthening blood vessels against circulatory diseases is an important nutrient attribute of soya milk, which arises from its rich source of Omega-3 and Omega-6 unsaturated fatty acid composition and the power phyto-antioxidants in the soya milk. These anti-oxidants and unsaturated fats bind to blood vessels linings and protect the blood cells from attack by toxic free radicals that may build up in the body tissues.

Soya milk provides generally lower calories consumption and therefore promoting weight loss because soya milk has lower sugar content 7 grams per100g compared to 12 grams in dairy milk.

Prostate cancer prevention by soya milk comes from the combined effects of its rich phyto-antioxidants and rich source of phytoestrogens that reduce excessive testosterone levels which could cause prostate cancer.

Phytoestrogens help post-menopausal women with an alternative oestrogen source to make postmenopausal women feel good with the extra oestrogen from the phytoestrogen effects.

Phytoestrogens also promote calcium intake into the body, into the bone tissues so preventing osteoporosis.

## 1.1I: INDUSTRIAL PRODUCTION TECHNOLOGY OF SOYA MILK

Soya milk became a traditionally produced food for the Chinese people some 2000 years ago when they developed a simple traditional method to produce it from water treated soya bean. The traditional soya milk producing method has remained the same since then being adapted and only a little modified by modern industrial uses. The production process starts with the making of a soya milk base from the soya bean as follows:

1. At a selected temperature of choice, soya beans are soaked in water for 4 to 12 hours depending on the temperature.
2. The soaked soya beans are next subjected to grinding into a mash by an electric grinder (originally the Chinese used stone to grind) with water being added so as to form a colloidal liquid from the ground pulp.
3. The slurry formed is cooked in a commercial steam injected vessel, making the soya milk.
4. The soya milk is next separated from fibrous *okara* by filtration or by use of industrial centrifuge.
5. The soya milk has an off flavour from the beans and that is removed next by processes that inhibit the enzyme lipo oxygenase that causes the off flavour of the milk.

6. A modified processing method now uses treating at high temperature the soya bean with sodium bicarbonate which destroys the off flavour forming enzyme lipo oxygenase; grinding until a colloid forms without the enzyme activity.
7. Water is next added to the colloid in sufficient amount to make the desired soya milk up to the required standard.
8. Flavours are then added to improve taste of the soya milk; suitable edible oil is added to improve taste giving rich appearance and flavour.

## 1.2 HONEY MAKING FROM FLOWER NECTAR BY BEES:

Natural honey is made by bees from the best nectar of many different types of flowers that are identified by the bees. It is rich in vitamins and antioxidants as shown in table 1.2.

Table 1.2: Honey nutrients composition:

| CONSTITUENT | PER 100g |
|---|---|
| PROTEIN 18 AMINO ACIDS (PROLINE mostly) | 0.5g |
| SUGARS :FRUCTOSE 38% GLUCOSE 31%, DISACCHARIES 9%, sucrose, maltose, isomaltose; oligosacch 4.2%, erlose, panose | 81.0g |
| FAT | trace |
| FIBRE | trace |
| SODIUM | trace |
| OTHER SALTS, minerals; calcium, iron, zinc, potassium, phosphorous, magnesium, selenium, chromium, manganese | trace |
| FLAVONOIDS (ANTIOXIDANTS) | present |
| GLUCOSE OXIDASE & invertase | present |
| HYDROGEN PEROXIDE, acetic, butanoic, lactic, citric, succinic, malic, formic, gluconic & pyroglutamic acid | present |
| VITAMIN B, C, B6, FOLATE | present |

## 1.2 THE HEALTH BENEFITS OF NATURAL PURE HONEY FROM BEES

Honey originates from God's creation of the promised land for Abraham (Genesis 12) and was one of the sweet things that Joshua and Caleb saw in the promised land when the Israeli children were still in the wilderness arguing on whether to go forward and take it or go back to Egypt from where they had suffered persecution (Numbers 13: 30). Joshua and Caleb discovered that the promised-land was a land full of 'milk and honey' in their faithful report to Moses and as testimony of their own faith in God (Numbers 13: 20; 26-30; Numbers 13: 23; Numbers 14: 24). In Proverbs 24: 13, our Almighty God Himself tells us very clearly: "My son, eat thou honey because it is good: and the honeycomb, which is sweet to thy taste:" Therefore God created honey for us in a very special way for a reason; the reason for our health benefits. The Biblical diet of goat milk and honey is well known in the scriptures together with the pomegranate fruit we mentioned earlier (Numbers 13: 23 – 24).

**The formation of natural honey by bees and the traditional health benefits of honey:** Bees were naturally created by God to always get to the best good looking flowers where the bees collect the nectar to make the honey. The biochemistry of flower nectar is now known; it contains almost 600 natural compounds that make honey that special and beneficial to health. Among these compounds, honey contains flavonoids antioxidants that prevent some cancers and heart disease. Honey also reduces stomach ulcers and gastroenteritis. Antibacterial and antifungal actions of honey are also known to come from the enzyme that bees add to form hydrogen peroxide in the honey. Ancient athletes are known to have used honey and dried figs to enhance performance and therefore it is prudent for modern athletes to try this natural remedy as I earlier mentioned its possible contribution to my own athletic performance in Chapter 2. Buckwheat honey especially has been shown to be a good cure for coughs. Honey is also known to strengthen the immune system for people. It enhances performance endurance and reduces muscle fatigue for athletes. The chemical composition of typical natural honey is shown in table 1.2.

1.3 HOW TO FARM HONEY BEES: Farming honey bees and selling honey can be very profitable business if you set it up professionally. i. Attend a brief beekeeping course as given by your nearest local bee experts. ii. Network with a friend who keeps bees. iii. Choose a suitable area on your farm where there is plenty of flowering plants (such as sunflowers or flowering sweet fruit trees which you can grow yourself deliberately near the bees) so as to provide bees with nectar and pollen. iv. Get your SEED BEES from your local friend beekeeper or order online from registered APIARIES. To start good bee farming you may need about £500 or US$800 approximately and increase productivity scale according to your own farming capacity. You can buy pre-packed bees and queens; each pack weighing about 2kg. v. EQUIPMENT: Includes hives; brood chamber; queen excluder; honey cupers; feeders; inner and outer covers for weather protection. vi. Beekeeper's protective gear: veil and long gloves. Then go farming and enjoy the bees working for you!

REFERENCE: Patent number 20090317533 (Method for production of soya milk): 24 December 2009: Inventors: Martin Herrmann and D.E. Wundsdorf: IPC8CLASS: 8823C1100FI; USPC CLASS: 426598; and; www. fao.org(2003). Eden Foods: Soya beverage manufacturing process. M.I.Clinton: 1997.

www.soya.be/benefits-soy-milk.php May 2013.

P.C. Molan (1992). The antibacterial activity of honey. Bee World 1992: 73 (1): 5 – 28. www.lancashirebeekeepers.org.uk

www.care2.com:Diana Harrington August 2012

# CHAPTER SIX

## HEALTHY RED COLOURED AND BLUE COLOURED FRUIT JUICES AND MIXTURES

1. POMEGRANATE JUICE Table1.Typical nutrients per 100 ml of the juice

| NUTRIENT | TYPICAL VALUE PER 100 ML | |
|---|---|---|
| PROTEIN | 0.1g | |
| SUGARS | 9.2g | |
| FAT (UNSATURATES) | trace | |
| FIBRE | 0.1g | |
| SALT EQUIVALENT | trace | |
| VITAMIN C | 30mg | |
| BOTH THE COMMERCIAL FRESH JUICE (1). & THE COMMERCIAL PHENOLIC COMPOUNDS | CONCENTRATE (2) HAVE ANTIOXIDANT ACTIVITY AS SHOWN HERE | |
| | 1.FRESH COMMERCIAL CONCENTRATE | 2. |
| 1$^{ST}$ GROUP PANTHOCYANINS | JUICE FRESH | JUICE CONCENTRATE |
| e.g. delphinidin 3, 4 glucoside | 6.11g | 2.11g |
| Cynidins 2, 5 diglucoside | 7.14g | 3.14g |
| TOTAL Anthocyanins | 35.74g | 16.19g |
| 2$^{ND}$ GROUP GALLAGYL TANNINS | | |
| e.g. punicalagan B | 42.13g | 43.49g |
| TOTAL Gallagyl tannins | 156.17g | 187.88g |
| 3$^{RD}$ GROUP ELLAGIC ACID DERIVATIVES | | |
| e.g. ellagic acid glucoside | 8.32g | 9.13g |
| TOTAL Ellagic derivatives | 12.11g | 26.40g |
| 4$^{TH}$ GROUP OTHER HYDROLYSABLE TANNINS e.g galloyl glucose | 4.9g | 6.55g |
| Total hydrolysable tannins | 41.73g | 55.86g |

Some Israeli Biochemists showed that pomegranate juice contains the highest antioxidant activity than any other fruit juices and it exceeds antioxidant activity of red grapes. Taking pomegranate juice daily is known to improve heart health and to strengthen man's libido and overall vitality (Song of Solomon 6:

9-11), preventing many types of cancers including prostate cancer.

Pomegranate is a fruit whose popularity originates from Biblical times (Haggai 2: 19) and some Iranians claim that it is the forbidden fruit pomegranate that tempted Eve in the Garden of Eden. Pomegranate indeed must have been a very important fruit flourishing in the Garden of Eden (Genesis). The health benefits of pomegranate are also described in more detail in Chapter 7. The health benefits originating from tannins in pomegranate are associated mainly with the pomegranate peel that was used in ancient times to treat anaemia, dysentery, intestinal worms, inflammation, bleeding, swellings and diarrhoea. Pomegranate fruit is also known to increase man's fertility. Antioxidant effects or toxins destruction effects and anti-cancer effects of pomegranate peel extracts have been described by P.S. Negi et al. Antibacterial effects and antioxidant effects of pomegranate peel were also shown by Negi and Jayaprakasha.

2. CRANBERRY JUICE

Table 2: Typical nutrients per 100 ml of juice

| NUTRIENT | TYPICAL VALUES PER 100 ML |
|---|---|
| PROTEIN | trace |
| SUGARS | 12.4g |
| FAT (SATURATES) | trace |
| FIBRE | trace |
| SODIUM | trace |
| SALTS EQUIVALENT | trace |
| VITAMIN C | 25.0mg |
| A-TYPE PROANTHOCYANIDINS | effective against urinary tract bacteria at 60ug/ml |

Cranberry juice is known to keep the urinary tract healthy through the effect of A type-Proanthocyanidins found only in

Cranberry juice but not in grape or other juices. Preliminary clinical trials are reported have shown some improvement on memory for dementia victims who were regularly given cranberry juice.

Cranberry juice contains large amounts of salicylic acid, an aspirin like compound and therefore those allergic to aspirin should not drink the juice.

HEALTH ALERT: Cranberry juice also contains large amounts of oxalates that are known to promote kidney stones. Therefore because of the potential hazards of oxalates on kidneys, too much cranberry juice should be avoided.

Cranberries reduce low density lipoprotein (LDL) oxidation and improve high density lipoprotein levels HDL and therefore reducing stroke risks and keeping healthy the cardiovascular system. The effects of cranberry extracts in giving health benefits to the urinary tract are described fully by Howell.

3. TOMATO JUICE: Table 3: Typical nutrients per 100 ml of juice

| NUTRIENT | TYPICAL VALUES PER 100 ML |
|---|---|
| PROTEIN | 0.6g |
| SUGARS | 3.9g |
| FAT | trace |
| FIBRE | 0.1g |
| SODIUM | 0.2g |
| SALTS EQUIVALENT | 0.6g |
| SIGNIFICANT VITAMINS CONTENT | |
| VITAMIN C | 18.3mg |
| NIACIN | 0.7mg |
| RIBOFLAVIN | 0.04mg |
| VITAMIN E | 0.7mg |
| MINERALS | 0.1g |
| VOLATILE ACIDS | 0.4g |

Tomato juice extracts contain antioxidants that include lycopene, vitamin E and beta-carotene. These antioxidants and other phytonutrients from tomato juice have been shown to lower blood pressure. Lycopene is believed to act by destroying the toxic free radicals that can cause cell damage if they accumulate. Lycopene and beta carotene antioxidants combined may contribute to the anti-prostate cancer effect of tomatoes. Lycopene is the red pigment that makes tomatoes red when ripe and it is also being chemically extracted in bulk as a preservative or natural colorant to other foods and juices or pharmaceuticals. Tomato extracts have also been shown to boost immunity, good for the heart, promote healthy hair, improve the eyes and contain chromium that helps improve diabetes control.

4. RED GRAPES JUICE: Table 4: Typical nutrients per 100 ml of juice

| NUTRIENT | YPICAL VALUES PER 100 ML |
|---|---|
| PROTEIN | 0.1g |
| SUGARS | 15.5g |
| FAT (SATURATES) | trace |
| FIBRE | trace |
| SODIUM | trace |
| SALTS EQUIVALENT | trace |

Red grapes concentrated juice caused increased antioxidant effects on LDL in both haemodialysis patients and normal people, also causing increased HDL, this being beneficial to increased cardiovascular health. Red grapes also have anticancer antioxidants namely resveratrol (a stilbene antioxidant), catechins and proanthocyanidins, as other antioxidants. These natural compounds are associated with good antioxidant effectiveness against colon cancer, prostate and breast cancer.

After the 40 days and 40 nights of the destruction of the earth and all other inhabitants by the Biblical floods, Noah became the first farmer (husbandsman) to plant grapes in a large scale vineyard and he got rather exceedingly happy of the results of his labour! (Genesis 9: 20 – 21).

5. RED GUAVA JUICE: Table 5: Typical nutrients per 100g of fruit: Modified from USDA Nutrient data base

| NUTRIENT | TYPICAL VALUES PER 100g |
|---|---|
| VITAMIN C | 228 mg (More than orange with 69mg) |
| POTASSIUM | 417mg (More than banana) |
| VITAMIN A | 624 IU |
| FOLIC ACID | 49ug |
| COPPER | 0.230mg |
| MANGANESE | 0.150mg |
| PHOSPHOROUS | 11mg |
| PHYTOCHEMICALS | + + |
| FIBRE | 5.4g |
| BETA CAROTENE | 374ug (Present as antioxidant) |
| LUTEIN | Present as antioxidant |
| CRYPTOXANTHIN | 0 ug |
| LYCOPENE | 5204ug (Antioxidant against cancer) |
| CALORIES | 68 KCAL |
| SUGARS (ARBOHYDRATES) | 14.3g |
| CALCIUM | 18mg |
| MAGNESIUM | 22mg |

The red coloured guava has more potent antioxidants against cancer than the yellow, green or white. Guava is good at preventing breast cancer and gargling guava juice is known to treat toothache and gum disease through the anti-gingivitis action of the folates in guava. The high concentration of vitamin C enables guava effective to treat gum bleeding; guava also treats diarrhoea and dysentery and is good at treating common colds coughs. Guava juice is also known to control epilepsy, convulsions and to heal wounds externally, reducing skin aging if one washes the skin with the unripe fruit and guava leaves liquid extract and treating oral ulcers. Guava is a healthy fruit for those who want to lose weight, eating the fruit with its low calories but rich protein and rich antioxidants for protection against diseases.

BLUE BERRIES JUICE: Table 6: Typical nutrients per 100 ml of juice

| NUTRIENT | TYPICAL VALUES PER 100 ML |
|---|---|
| VITAMIN A | 79.9 IU |
| VITAMIN C | 14.4mg |
| VITAMIN E | 0.8mg |
| VITAMIN K | 28.6ug |
| POTASSIUM | 114mg |
| FOLATE | 45ug |
| VITAMIN B12 | 8.9ug |
| CALORIES | 84.4 KCAL |
| SUGARS | 21.4g |
| PROTEIN | 1.2g |
| DIETARY FIBRE | 3.6g |
| OMEGA 3 FATTY ACIDS | 85.8mg |
| OMEGA 6 FATTY ACIDS | 130mg |
| THIAMIN | 0.1mg |
| RIBOFLAVIN | 0.1mg |
| NIACIN | 0.6mg |
| VITAMIN B6 | 0.1mg |
| CHOLINE | 8.9mg |
| BETAINE | 0.3mg |

Blueberries have shown to reduce by over 30% the risk of cardiovascular disease for women who regularly daily take blueberries and strawberries in their diet. A blueberries diet was also shown to improve brain health through strengthened motor coordination, protecting against aging and against Azheimer's disease.. Blueberries diet helps weight reduction even the berries are eaten with fat. Blueberries, together with cherries and strawberries help in getting rid of gout.

HEALTH ALERT: Blueberries contain salicylates and therefore may need to be avoided if one is being prescribed anticoagulants; check with your Doctor if you are under medication before you take the blueberries into diet.

Antioxidants in blueberries include polyphenols that give the blue colour to the blue berry and vitamin C which works as powerful antioxidant that promotes a strong immune system; prevents gum diseases, cancers and supports a healthy cardiovascular system with healthy blood capillaries as well as promoting strong collagen formation. Blueberries antioxidant phytonutrients are five major categories as anthocyanins that include: (malvidins, elphinidins, elargonidins, cyanidins, peonidins); hydroxycinnamic acids (caffeic acid, ferulic acid, and coumaric acid), hydroxybenzoic acids (coumaric acid, gallic acid, and procathuic acid), flavonols (kaempferol, quercetin, myricetin) and other phenol related phytonutrients (pterostilbene, resveratrol). These complex groups of antioxidants therefore make blueberries a very good defence food and drink against many diseases including several cancers and breast cancer.

6. STRAWBERRIES JUICE: Table 7: Typical nutrients per 100 ml of juice

| NUTRIENT | TYPICAL VALUES PER 100 ML |
|---|---|
| VITAMIN C | 84.67mg |
| MANGANESE | 0.56mg |
| FIBRE | 2.88g |
| FOLATE | 34.56ug |
| IODINE | 12.96ug |
| POTASSIUM | 220.32mg |
| MAGNESIUM | 18.72mg |
| VITAMIN K | 3.17ug |
| OMEGA 3 FATS | 0.09g |

Strawberries are known to be packed with antioxidants and anti-inflammatory phytonutrients. There are approximately six groups of these complex compounds in strawberries as follows: anthocyanins for example: (cyaninidins, pelargonidins), flavonols including: (procyanidins, catechins, gallocatechins, epicatechins, kaempferol, quercetin), hydroxybenzoic acid (ellagic acid, gallic acid, vanillic acid, salicylic acid), hydroxycinnamic acid (cinnamic acid, coumaric acid, caffeic acid, ferulic acid), tannins (ellagitannins, gallotanins) and stilbenes (resveratrol). These antioxidants and phytonutrients make strawberries very good protectors of good health by destroying cancer causing radicals from the body, boosting the immune system, protecting the cardiovascular system; being anti-diabetes together with many other antioxidant effects similar to those of blueberries. The other important nutrients of strawberry juice are shown in table 7 in this chapter.

7. PRUNE (DRIED PLUM) JUICE CONCENTRATE: Table 8: Typical nutrients per 100ml of juice

| NUTRIENT | TYPICAL VALUES PER 100 ML |
|---|---|
| PROTEIN | 0.7g |
| SUGARS | 13.0g |
| OTHER CARBOHYDRATES | 3.8g |
| FAT (UNSATURATES) | 0.1g |
| SATURATED FATS | trace |
| FIBRE | 1.2g |
| SODIUM | trace |
| SALTS EQUIVALENT | trace |
| VITAMIN K | 25.88ug |
| FIBRE | 3.09g |
| POTASSIUM | 318.12mg |

Prunes are actually dried plums and when dried and wrinkly, they are not attractive and are wrongly suspected of causing constipation. Plums have a high content of antioxidants and the dried prune is a high source of fibre that prevents constipation. The antioxidant effect of prunes is to lower cholesterol and the plum juice decreases incidence of colon cancer. More nutrients of dried plum juice are shown in table 8 in this chapter.

REFERENCES: A. Cassidy, K.J. Mukamai, L. Liu, M. Franz, H. Eliassen and E. Rimm (2013). Circulation: Journal of the American Heart Association: 127: 188 – 196.

A.A. Bertelli and D.K. Das: J. Cardiovascular. Pharmacology 54 (6) 468 – 476: December 2009.

A.B.Howell.(2002). Critical Review of Food Science Nutrition 42: (3 suppl): 273 – 278.

J.A. Joseph, N.A. Denisova, G. Arendash, M. Gordon, D. Diamond, B. Shukitt-Hale and D. Morgan (2003, 1999): Nutritional Neuroscience 2003: 6: 153 – 162; Journal of Neuroscience 1999: 19(18): 8114 – 8121.

D. Bhowmik, K.P.S. Kumar, S. Paswan and S. Srivastiva: May 2012; www.phytojournal.com.Journal of Pharmacognosy and Phytochemistry: 1 (1) pp 35 - 43: (ISSN 2278 – 4136 online.

L.S. Adam, S. Phung, N. Yee, N.P. Seeram, L. Li and S. Chen (2010): Cancer Research: May 1: 70 (9): 3594 – 3605.

R.Castilla, A. Echarri, F.Davalos, H. Cerrato, J.L Ortega, M.F. Tereul, D. Lucas, D. Gomez-Coronado, J. Ortuno and M.A. Lascuncio: American Journal of Clinical Nutrition: 84 (1) pp 252 – 262; July 2006).

P.S. Negi, G.K. Javaprakasha and B.S. Jena. (Food Chemistry:80 (3) March 2003: pp 393 – 397).

P.S.Negi and G.K Jayaprakasha (Journal of Food Science 68: (4) May 2003 : pp 1473 - 1477; P.S.Negi and G.K. Jayaprakasha).

www.nutrition-and-you.com:May.2013.

www.organicfacts.netMay 2013

www.whfoods.com May 2013. ; www.cranberryinstitute.org

www.nim.nih.gov/medlineplus US National Library of Health.

Chetali Samanti: www.spiceflair.com September 14, 2012.

# CHAPTER SEVEN
## PURE MIXED TROPICAL AND OTHER FRUITS JUICE
1. TYPICAL MIXTURE OF BANANAS MANGOES ORANGES LEMON PINEAPPLE MELON APPLE PEACH TOMATO AND POMEGRANATE

This type of tropical mixed fruit juice is rich in the multiple nutrients that come with each different type of fruit as listed in the fruits mixture list (Tables 1.1 and 1.2). A typical banana is rich in potassium and flavonoids, vitamins and antioxidants that prevent several types of cancers.

Table 1: Mixed Tropical commercial fruits juice nutrients table:

| NUTRIENT | TYPICAL VALUE PER 100 ML |
|---|---|
| PROTEIN | TRACE |
| SUGARS | 5.3g |
| FATS | NIL |
| FIBRE | TRACE |
| SODIUM | TRACE |
| VITAMIN C | 30mg |
| OTHER ANTIOXIDANTS AND VITAMINS | As summarised in the table 1.1 for all fruits |

1.1 BANANA FRUIT HEALTH BENEFITS: In all the 10 fruits juice mixture illustrated in table 1.1 below, banana juice contributes the most sugar (carbohydrates) nutrient at 22.4g per 100g of fruit. Of these sugars, banana pulp consists of predominantly **fructose and sucrose sugars** which are easily digestible and therefore suitable for a busy, energetic or athletic lifestyle where a lot of energy is required. Banana contributes also the highest content of potassium at 385mg per 100g of fruit topping all the other 9 fruits of the mixture on potassium nutrient. Potassium is very beneficial to active lifestyle by regulating bps, keeping people safe against the otherwise adverse effects of too much sodium from dietary salts. Potassium is needed for normal heart, kidney and other organs to function properly. Deficiency in potassium results in muscle crumbs for example and cancer, arthritis, heart disease may occur if potassium supply is low. Fatigue and muscle weakness may also occur if potassium is not enough from fluid intakes. Athletes therefore will need adequate potassium in their rehydration drinks to keep fit and to achieve top performance.

Of the 10 fruits in the typical commercial mixture (table 1.1), banana fruit has the highest amount of the vitamins pyridoxine at 0.367g per 100g, riboflavin at 0.073g and the third largest amount of folates at 20 mcg per 100g. Therefore banana contributes considerably to the overall antioxidants nutrients in the fruit juice mixture. **Vitamin B6** (Pryridoxine) is required daily by the body to produce antibodies and red blood cells. It is water soluble and is part of the Vitamin B complex. Therefore the banana fruit is a good natural source for boosting antibody production and red blood cells for example soon after an injury bleeding and an infection. Vitamin B6 is a precursor coenzyme for over sixty other coenzymes needed in the body for healthy metabolic functions; such as by combating several diseases and producing serotonin in the brain for happiness and well-being. Overall, Vitamin B6 is important for diuretic properties; cardiovascular well-being, may reduce epilectic seizures, produces brain stimulating chemicals, protein and fat metabolism, converting tryptophan to niacin, producing anti-aging nucleic acids, reducing asthma and strengthening nerve functions. Riboflavin is needed in the body for similar functions to those of Vitamin B6 and is required daily in the body.

Adequate amounts of folate are required daily for healthy foetal development, producing red blood cells, preventing heart disease, has anti-aging effects keeping the brain young and keeps people happy working against depression.

Banana also contains the highest amount at 1.0ug of the essential trace element selenium. Selenium is an antioxidant that is necessary to keep men fit; it supports healthy eyes and healthy hair but is only good in low trace amounts. Too much selenium may turn to toxicity and unnecessary supplements of selenium should be avoided.

Other vitamins and nutrients present in banana fruit are B-carotene also with antioxidant beneficial effects, vitamin A, vitamin C, vitamin E and vitamin K.

Magnesium is also present in the highest amount at 27mg per 100g in the banana fruit more than the other 9 fruits (table 1.1), and phosphorous at third largest amount of 22mg per 100g of the fruit. Low magnesium intake by men may cause aging, muscle weakness, atherosclerosis, diabetes and increased risk of prostate cancer. Phosphorous forms predominantly part of the bone tissue in which 85% of the body's phosphorous is found. It is important for strong bones and teeth, combining with calcium and vitamin D in the bone matrix. In all the other body tissues, phosphorous may well work in synergy with potassium promoting cellular tissue activities and metabolic activities to potassium.

Dietary fibre and fats are found in the banana fruit; and some calcium, copper and iron and low sodium content.

**1.2 MANGO FRUIT HEALTH BENFITS:** Mango fruit contains the highest amounts of Vitamin A at 765 IU per 100g, and Vitamin C at 27.7 mg per 100g and Vitamin E at 1,12mg per 100g, more than the other nine fruits in the juice mixture. Nutrients in mango fruit have been shown recently to protect against several types of cancers; including cancer of the breast, the colon, leukaemia and the prostate cancer.

**Vitamin A** health benefits include functions as coenzyme for several enzymes for tissue metabolism in the body; and it has both preventive and therapeutic uses on several diseases. Vitamin A strengthens the body immune system to combat infections and can prevent the HIV virus from spreading in the body. Vitamin A stops cancer from spreading by inhibiting DNA replication in the cancer cells. When applied to already existing cancer cells, vitamin A stops the cancer cells from growing. However recently a paradox effect of pre-existing vitamin A on HIV has been found to actually promote the spread of the HIV virus and therefore vitamin A is not given to such HIV carriers. Vitamin A is also used in eye drops to restore moisture back into the eye.

**Vitamin C** is one of the most powerful antioxidants in mango juice and it gives the health benefits of combating many diseases. Recently vitamin C was found to be good at reducing bps and protecting the heart and the cardiovascular system. Vitamin C also helps prevent asthma and cancer. Biochemically as a potent antioxidant, Vitamin C removes toxic free radicals from tissues and the blood, providing a healthier life and well-being to the individual. Vitamin C reduces cellular DNA damage in a crucial step to prevent the onset of cancers. Supplement of vitamin C is known to effectively protect against toxic smoke inhalations. Vitamin C supplement is also shown by researchers to protect the body against toxins released by people during vigorous exercise. Therefore it is a good healthy practice for everyone doing vigorous exercise, athletics or other sports to take a daily supplement of vitamin C as it gives a win win effect by also protecting the cardiovascular system and against gastric cancer.

Vitamin E is known to be protective against neurological diseases such as Azheimer's and diabetes. Its other name is tocopherol and it has antioxidant properties and is fat soluble. It is available only through diet intake of the vitamin E containing foods. Vitamin E is good for skin care and also nourishes the hair and is good for cardiovascular circulation around the skin preventing what is called sun strokes and it also alleviates fatigue.

Other nutrients in mango are all listed in table 1.1 and these include sugars, protein and dietary fibre and several nutrient minerals.

1.2 ORANGES HEALTH BENEFITS: Orange fruit contributes, out of the ten fruits (table 1.1), the highest amount of thiamine vitamin in the fruit juice mixture with 0.103mg per 100g. Thiamine vitamin B1 is an important component of the B complex vitamins which is crucial for larger carbohydrate breakdown to the glucose sugar body cells can use. Orange also has the third largest amount of pantothenic acid at 0.250g per 100g in table 1.1 showing the ten fruits. Orange also has the largest content of vitamin C at the same level with lemon each at 53mg per 100g (table 1.1).

Thiamine vitamin B1 is part of the enzyme complex that breaks down sugars to produce energy for the body. The energy for a good athlete and sportsman comes from the direct metabolic actions of vitamin B1 in association with a good dietary balance with other vitamins in the body. Heart function is also known to be improved by vitamin B1, as much as the vitamin is also known to reduce the aging process and to prevent Azheimer's disease. Thiamine is also known to be good at improving the memory and improving overall cardiac function.

**Pantothenic acid vitamin B5** an important vitamin known to prevent stress and anxiety and keeps people happy and healthy; it improves immunity, checks out aging by improving overall vitality; it is a well-known one solution for a number of diseases and therefore it is only wise to take suitable daily supplement of it. Other nutrients are also present in orange in moderate amounts as listed in table 1.1. Orange also has the highest amount of calcium at 40mg per 100g, out of all the ten fruit mixtures. **Calcium** is needed for healthy bone and teeth formation.

Orange also contains a group of very good antioxidant phytochemicals namely: **hesperetin, naringon** and **naringen;** these being flavonoids. Naringen is known to be a good antioxidant; a free radicals remover and to be anti-inflammatory and as an immune system modulator.

1.4 LEMON HEALTH BENEFITS: Lemon is a low calories fruit. Lemon has the highest amount of iron 8mg, vitamin C 53mg, pyridoxine 0.8g and dietary fibre 2.8g per 100g. The health benefits of vitamin C have already been described in section 1.1. **Iron** is required in red blood cells production together with the build-up of haemoglobin and muscle myoglobin both being proteins of oxygen transport in the blood and in the muscles respectively. Iron deficiency may cause fatigue and general body weakness. Therefore a top class sportsman must have sufficient body iron to prevent premature fatigue during intense competitions for example.

Pyridoxine is vitamin B6 which is important for serotonin production, reduces heart disease and it converts tryptophan to serotonin, being called a vitamin of remembering sweet dreams. Pyridoxal phosphate comes from vitamin B6 and has important metabolic functions in the body as a coenzyme for fat, glucose, amino acids and histamine metabolism and overall gene expression within body cells.

Dietary fibre is required for good food digestion so as to improve nutrients for uptake into the blood. Fibres in digestion may also lower cholesterol uptake into the blood stream.

1.5 PINEAPPLE HEALTH BENEFITS: Pine apple contains the third largest amount of Vitamin C in table 1.1 and the largest amount of manganese at 0.927mg per 100g.

Manganese is very essential for bone structure and bone strength, forming connective tissue, production of sex hormones, regulating thyroid functions and antioxidant effect removing tree radicals from the body. Manganese is also a metabolic co-factor for the enzyme superoxide dismutase a very strong free radicals remover and cofactor for enzymes in the regulation of sugar metabolism. Pineapple also produces the proteolytic enzyme called Bromelain which promotes anti-inflammation, anti-cancer and anti-clotting catalytic activity within the cells and tissues. Vitamin C in pineapple and other fruits also promotes collagen biosynthesis. Therefore most antioxidants work at DNA or mRNA level of cellular control to prevent diseases.

**1.6 HEALTH BENEFITS OF MELON FRUIT:** Melon is also a low calories fruit but is the richest with Vitamin A content of 3382 IU and the second largest amount of magnesium at 18mg per 100g. Vitamin A is also a powerful antioxidant, good for vision. Melon is rich in flavonoids; B-carotene, lutein, zea xanthin and crypto xanthin which all protect the cells and body tissues against free radical damage; protect against prostate cancer, colon cancer and breast cancer; against endometrial, lung and pancreatic cancers. Vitamin A is also called retinoid is good for the immune system and healthy skin in addition to giving good eye vision. Out of the ten fruits (table 1.1) melon produces the most B-carotene at 2020ug per 100g.

Magnesium is required for healthy digestion of food, good metabolic control of sugars metabolism, maintaining a healthy heart and keeping bones healthy. It is a powerful antioxidant and reduces the risk of cancer developing.

**1.7 APPLE FRUIT HEALTH BENEFITS:** Apple juice is rich in phyto nutrients and contains powerful antioxidants to combat many diseases. Apple nutrients give good well-being to people because they include the antioxidants flavonoids and polyphenols with total antioxidant value of 5900 TE per 100g. The flavonoids in apple include quercetin, epicatechin, procyanidin; in addition to large amounts of tartaric acid which also has antioxidant effects. Apple also contains B-crypto xanthin and lutein zea xanthin as other very potent antioxidants.

**1.8 PEACH FRUIT HEALTH BENEFITS:** Peach contains a very rare antioxidant lycopene, and has the largest content of lutein zea xanthin and crypto xanthin (table 1.1). Peach is also rich in potassium and together with these antioxidants, peach has great health benefits. **Lutein zea xanthin** is also known to improve eye vision. **Lycopene** is an antioxidant that prevents formation of harmful by products from metabolic pathways by removal free radicals. **Cryptoxanthin** is a carotenoid derivative type of antioxidant; it may give anti-ageing benefits, protecting against heart disease and cancers.

1.9 HEALTH BENEFITS OF TOMATO: Tomato is the lowest calories fruit with only 18 calories, out of the ten in table 1.1 as it has only 3.9g sugar per 100g compared to 22.84g for banana. Tomato is rich in phosphorous and vitamin K. **Vitamin K** is a bone builder and heart protector. Tomato also has high potassium content and tomato also contains a patented content of lycopene antioxidant. Vitamin K promotes blood clotting through carboxylation. Vitamin K may have the same antioxidant potency as vitamin C and E or may have a synergistic effect to these two.

1.10 HEALTH BENEFITS OF POMEGRANATE: Pomegranate is associated with enhancing man's vitality and performance. Pomegranate contains **pulicalagin polypeptide antioxidant** that reduces heart disease *risk*. Antioxidant total capacity is 2341 umol TE per 100g and the pomegranate antioxidant is known to protect against prostate cancer and diabetes; making all men happy for that! Pomegranate also contains ellargic acid, gallic acid and anthocyanins; all these antioxidants being associated with overall man's vitality and virility since the creation of man by God in the Garden of Eden (Genesis 1).

Table 1.1: Major nutrients in 10 selected fruits for a mixed commercial fruit juice per 100g of the original fruit. 1= Banana, 2 = Mango, 3 = Orange, 4 = Lemon, 5 = Pineapple, 6 = Melon, 7 = Apple, 8 = Peach, 9 = Tomato, 10 = Pomegranate:

IN THE FRUIT JUICEMIXTURE, EACH INDIVIDUAL FRUIT IS CONTRIBUTING ITS OWN SPECIAL NUTRIENTS: ug = mcg = micro. g

| FRUIT | 1 | 2 | 3 | 4 | 5 | 6 | 7 | 8 | 9 | 10 |
|---|---|---|---|---|---|---|---|---|---|---|
| Nutrient | Value | Value | V | V | Value | V | V | Value | Value | Value |
| Sugars | 22.84g | 17g | 11.75g | 9.32g | 13.52g | 8.5g | 13.8g | 9.54g | 3.9g | 18.7g |
| Protein | 1.09g | 0.5g | 0.94g | 1.10g | 0.54g | 0.84g | 0.26g | 0.91g | 0.9g | **1.67g** |
| Total Fat | 0.33g | 0.27g | 0.12g | 0.30g | 0.12g | 0.19g | 0.17g | 0.25g | 0.2g | 1.17g |
| Cholest | 0 | 0 | 0 | 0 | 0 | 0 | 0 | 0 | 0 | 0 |
| Di Fibre | 0.60g | 1.8g | 2.40g | **2.8g** | 1.40g | 0.9g | 2.4g | 1.5g | 1.2g | **4g** |
| **Vitamin** | | | | | | | | | | |
| Folates | 20ug | 10ug | 2.40ug | 11ug | 18ug | 21ug | 3ug | 4ug | 15ug | **38 ug** |
| Niacin | 0.665 mg | 0.584g | 0.282g | 0.10 mg | 0.50ug | 0.734g | 0.09 mg | 0.81 mg | 0.58 mg | 0.293 mg |
| Pantothenic acid | 0.334 mg | 0.160g | **0.250g** | 0.190g | - | 0.105ug | 0.46 mg | 0.153 mg | - | 0.135 mg |
| Pyridoxine | **0.367g** | 0.134 mg | 0.060 mg | **0.80g** | 0.112 mg | 0.072 mg | 0.04 mg | 0.025g | 0.08 mg | 0.075 mg |
| Riboflavin | **0.073g** | 0.057 mg | 0..040 mg | 0.02g | 0.018 mg | 0.036 mg | 0.026 mg | 0.031 mg | 0.037 mg | 0.053 mg |
| Thiamin | 0.031g | 0.031 mg | **0.106 mg** | 0.04g | 0.079 mg | 0.017 mg | 0.017 mg | 0.024 mg | 0.037 mg | 0.067 mg |
| Vitamin A | 60 IU | 765 IU | 225 IU | 22 IU | 58 IU | 338 2 IU | 54 IU | 326 IU | 233 IU | 0 |
| Vitamin C | 8.7mg | 27.7 mg | 53.2 mg | 53 mg | 47.18 mg | 36.7 mg | 4.6 mg | 6.6mg | 13mg | 10.2 mg |
| Vitamin E | 0.1mg | **1.12 mg** | 0.180 mg | 0.15 mg | 0.02 mg | 0.05 mg | 0.18 mg | 0.73 mg | 0.54 mg | 0.60 mg |
| *Vitamin K* | 0.5ug | 4.2ug | 0 | 0 | 0.07ug | 2.5ug | 2.2ug | 2.6ug | 7.9ug | **16.4ug** |

| Salts & Minerals | 1 | 2 | 3 | 4 | 5 | 6 | 7 | 8 | 9 | 10 |
|---|---|---|---|---|---|---|---|---|---|---|
| Sodium | 1mg | 2mg | 0 | 2mg | - | 1mg | 1mg | 0 | 5mg | 3mg |
| Potassium | 358 mg | 156 mg | 169 mg | 138 mg | 1mg | 2.07 mg | 107 mg | 190 mg | 237 mg | 236 mg |
| Calcium | 5mg | 10mg | 40mg | 26mg | 13mg | 9mg | 6 mg | 6mg | 10mg | 10mg |
| Copper | 0.078 mg | 0.110 g | 39ug | 37ug | 0..110 mg | 41ug | - | 0.068 mg | - | 0.158 mg |
| Iron | 0.26 mg | 0.13 mg | 0.10 mg | 8mg | 0.29 mg | 0.21 mg | 0.042 mg | 0.25 mg | 0.3mg | 0.3mg |
| Magnesium | 27mg | 9mg | 10mg | 8mg | 12mg | 18 mg | 5mg | 9mg | 11mg | 12mg |
| Manganese | 0.27 mg | 0.27 mg | 0.024 mg | 0.130 mg | 0.927 mg | 0.41 mg | - | 0.61 mg | 0.15 mg | 0.11 mg |
| Phosphorous | 22mg | - | - | - | 8mg | - | 11mg | 11mg | 24mg | 36mg |
| Selenium | 1.0ug | - | - | - | 0.1ug | - | - | - | - | - |
| Zinc | 0.15 mg | - | 0.08 mg | 0.06 mg | 0.12u g | - | 0.04 mg | - | 0.17 mg | 0.35 mg |
| B-Carotene | 35ug | - | - | - | - | 2020 ug | 27 ug | 449ug | - | - |
| B-Crypto Xanthin | trace | - | - | - | - | 1ug | 11ug | 101ug | - | - |
| Lutein zea xanthin | - | - | - | - | - | 26ug | 29ug | 123ug | - | - |
| Lycopene | - | - | - | - | - | - | - | 2573 ug | Present | - |

In great appreciation of His creation God said to the Israeli children; "For the Lord thy God bringeth thee into a good land, a land of brooks of water of fountains and depths that spring out of the valleys and hills.

A land of wheat and barley and vines and fig trees and pomegranates: a land of oil of olive and honey." (Deuteronomy 8: 7 – 8). Pomegranate was the best fruit that

God wanted us all to enjoy; together with grapes and fig tree representing all the other fruits; and healthy water to drink from the brooks and springs; up to today natural spring water is the best available natural water which is being harvested and bottled for commercial supplies world-wide. We all must thank God for all these precious gifts of life; the foods, fruits and water and our good health. The Biblical Shulamite woman particularly liked to see pomegranates budding in the garden because she knew their importance to her husband's vitality and performance (Song of Solomon 6:11).

## 1.11 THE DOMESTIC TECHNOLOGY OF PRODUCTION OF OWN FRESH FRUIT JUICE:

In the market there are many gadgets and machines designed to produce fresh fruit juice from the domestic kitchen; that is suitable for your own individual needs. The starting off point towards manufacturing our own favourite fruit juices is firstly identify an economically good source of the fruits at the lowest price possible. Then next; buy your chosen fruits in bulk that makes good economics compared to general market juices. Better also; farm your own fruits if you have a farm.

For oranges for example there is a wide range of machines specifically to make good orange juice only; ranging from small domestic to micro commercial and maxi commercial. One good type of micro commercial orange juice making machine is an Auto Feed type of machine in which the producer feeds into the machine, whole oranges without having to peel or cut to pieces. Such a machine clearly produces orange juice that is very rich in ALL the nutrients of fruit.

The best type of micro commercial orange mixed fruit juice machine is defined as the All Fruits Juicer and Vegetable

Juicer; as by its given name; can take in any type of fruit in a mixture and processes the fruit or vegetable without having to peel or cut to pieces the fruits or vegetables. This type of machine makes it possible to produce any type of fruit or vegetable juice you may want to. The machine produces mixed fruit juices that are rich in ALL the nutrients of the mixed fruits or mixed vegetables.

There is a wide market of these fruit juice and vegetable juice making machines to choose what you want as the best for your own needs; and to give yourself healthy fresh fruit juices and the healthy lifestyle of saving yourself some good cash during the process.

REFERENCES:

F.Poiroux-Gonord, L.P.R.Bidal, A.L. Fanciullino, H. Gautier, F. Lauri – Lopez and L. Urban (2010). Health benefits of vitamins and secondary metabolites of fruits and vegetables and prospects to increase their concentrations by agronomic approaches: Journal of Agricultural and Food Chemistry: 58 (23) 12065 – 12082. 10 November 2010.

Life Extension Magazine April 2008: Julius Goepp MD.
Natural News.com: Jonathan Benson: 19 FEBRUARY 2013.
www.nutrition-and-you.com:Poweryourdiet:Your.guide...
Organic Facts: www.organifacts.net.
www.cranberryinstitute.org.
Lycopene.com: Patented Natural Tomato Complex; by: Lyco Red 2011.
VITAMINSTUFF.COM May 2013: The Antioxidants Section.
Health &Wellness Library: www. nutriherb.net/*mineral or vitamin search*.html

# CHAPTER EIGHT
## HEALTHY HOT BEVERAGES

Healthy hot beverages are the dark cocoa and dark chocolates

1. COCOA: Typical nutrient values per 100 g of cocoa

| NUTRIENT | VALUE PER 100 g COCOA |
|---|---|
| PROTEIN | 23.1g |
| SUGAR | 0.0 |
| CARBOHYDRATE | 10.5g |
| UNSATURATED FATS | 8.3g |
| SATURATED FATS | 13.4g |
| FIBRE | 12.1g |
| SODIUM | 0.7g |
| OTHER SALT EQUIVALENT | 1.75g |
| ANTIOXIDANTS | 8% |

The health benefits of hot cocoa drink are similar but much more than those found in drinking hot chocolate. The original cocoa is produced from roasted and ground cocoa bean to produce a dark cocoa powder that has a bitter taste. The cocoa bean powder is then pressed to remove fat from it to make the dark fat-free cocoa powder from which various types of chocolates are produced by adding sweetener, sugar or honey. Recent research results show that it is healthier to drink the hot dark cocoa which is richer in antioxidants than chocolates. Cocoa drinkers can sweeten it for themselves with honey for example, for a healthy improved taste. The lesser the sugar in the dark brown cocoa powder the better and healthier. Cocoa is now regarded as an antioxidant itself containing a high amount of polyphenols; at 8% by weight of cocoa bean. The antioxidant capacity of cocoa comes mainly from its flavonol monomers; epicatechin and catechin and some procyanidins.

Chocolate drink, diet chocolate or dark chocolate are supplied according to individual groups of consumer preferences usually based on taste. But health benefits arise from nutrient quality; the darker the chocolate the healthier because of higher cocoa antioxidants in the hot drink.

## 2.0 CHOCOLATE

### 2.1 EU SOURCE DARK HOT CHOCOLATE: Typical nutrient value per 100g chocolate

| NUTRIENT | VALUE PER 100g (Approx. 6 cups hot drink) |
|---|---|
| CALORIES | 384.6 ( Approx. 60 calories per cup) |
| TOTAL FAT | 6.41g |
| CHOLESTEROL | 0 |
| TOTAL CARBOHYDRATE | 64.1g |
| DIETARY FIBRE | 6.41g |
| SUGARS | 44,87g |
| PROEIN | 12.82g |
| ANTIOXIDANTS | Very rich content |
| SODIUM | - |

Taken per cup therefore, the calories from one hot cup of black chocolate (table 2.1) are low; and health benefits of the antioxidants good effects of destroying body toxins, being ant-cancer far outweigh the calories problem in dark chocolate.

### 2.2 DIET EU BRAND HOT CHOCOLATE: Typical nutrient value per 100g chocolate

| NUTRIENT | VALUE PER 100g (Approx. 6 cups hot drink) |
|---|---|
| CALORIES | 166.6 (Approx. 25.99 calories per cup) |
| TOTAL FAT | 0 |
| CHOLESTEROL | 0 |
| TOTAL CARBOHYDRATE | 22.68g |
| DIETARY FIBRE | 6.6g |
| SUGARS | 12.6g |
| PROTEIN | 12.6g |
| ANTIOXIDANTS | Very rich content |
| SODIUM | 1.025g |

As shown in table (2.2), so called commercial diet chocolate has the lowest number of calories and is therefore suitable for the very rigorous weight watching individual who would like a daily drink of the diet chocolate.

2.3 A TYPICAL LOCAL UK COMMERCIAL HOT CHOCOLATE: Nutrient value per 100g chocolate of international standard quality (a Hypermarket retail source)

| NUTRIENT | VALUE PER 100g (Approx. 6 cups hot drink) |
|---|---|
| CALORIES | 412 (Approx. 67.5 calories per cup) |
| TOTAL FAT | 10.6g |
| CHOLESTEROL | 0 |
| TOTAL CARBOHYDRATE | 69.4 |
| DIETARY FIBRE | 5.2g |
| SUGARS | 55.9g |
| PROTEIN | 7.0g |
| ANTIOXIDANTS | Very rich content |
| SODIUM | - |

This UK local chocolate (table 2.3) has very similar calories content of about 60 per cup compared to the best known EU brand shown in table (2.2). This observation confirms that the particular Hypermarket selling the UK band in table 2.3 is keeping a very high standard of consumer supply with the chocolate that is close to the best EU standard shown in table 2.2. It is good to see traders being that loyal and honest to their consumers by keeping the highly valued international standards of quality products.

### 2.4 Another popular dark hot chocolate: Nutrient value per 100g chocolate (very popular international brand):

| NUTRIENT | VALUE PER 100g (Approx. 6 cups hot drink) |
|---|---|
| CALORIES | 762.79 (Approx. 119 per cup) |
| TOTAL FAT | 24.99g |
| TOTAL CARBOHYDRATE | 114.74g |
| DIETARY FIBRE | 3.85g |
| PROTEIN | 20.64g |
| ANTIOXIDANTS | Very rich content |
| SODIUM | - |

This very popular international brand shown in table 2.4 unfortunately has too many calories, 119 per cup, which do not come close to the best EU 60 calories per cup shown in table 2.2; but consumers still go for the popularity of the international brand shown in table 2.4 despite the high calories per cup. At certain times such as highly vigorous work or highly vigorous sports, people may actually choose the high calories drink over the low calories drink; so that it becomes purely personal choice sometimes against the health benefits of the lower calories. The important bottom line regarding all the chocolate commercial brands available is that all contain the basic antioxidants nutrient that help guard every regular chocolate drinker against cancers, whilst protecting the cardiovascular system as well. These benefits are described fully in the following paragraphs here.

The most highly recommended healthy hot chocolate drink is that which is prepared directly with hot water, and not whole milk, so as to avoid milk fat. It is also possible to choose sugar free hot chocolate brands or low calories brands.

Hot chocolate drink is rich in beneficial antioxidants; these can be defined as substances that reduce oxidative damage by oxygen group free radicals that may accumulate in the body as external toxins or products of bad metabolic processes. Research has shown that by destroying the toxic oxygen binding free radicals, chocolate antioxidants can prevent cancer, heart disease, premature ageing process and age related muscle degeneration. Therefore the hot chocolate antioxidants can indeed extend a man's life considerably as they prevent premature aging and diseases, as a blessing from God, similar to the long active life that Abraham was blessed with as written in the Holy Bible (Genesis 12).

Hot chocolate has three times more health benefits effect than tea or wine. Research scientists at Cornell University in the USA have reported that hot chocolate also contains gallic acid as additional antioxidants and gallic acid was shown to treat internal haemorrhage and albuminuria. The presence of albumin in urine indicates either diabetes or kidney damage. It was also shown that heating up the chocolate gives the added benefit of releasing more antioxidants into the boiling water. Chang Yong Lee of the Cornell University produced evidence demonstrating that it is more beneficial to drink hot chocolates than to eat it the commercial chocolate bars. This is because heated chocolate releases more flavonoids from the dark chocolate into the water. Flavonoids account for the chocolate dark colour and they are good at inducing release of nitric acid into the blood stream; causing relaxation of blood vessels. Nitric oxide also destroys parasitic organisms, virus infected cells and tumour cells. Drinking chocolate will also increase blood flow to the tissues, giving more vitality to man, helping to lower bps and at the same time promoting good heart health. The flavonoids in hot chocolate give the drink a beneficial "aspirin like" effect by preventing blood platelets from clamping up together; so effectively preventing the unhealthy hazards of thrombosis formations during circulation. The American Association for the Advancement of Science have reported that drinking hot chocolate also makes people think much better because of 'happy' stimulants being released into the brain. These stimulate increased blood flow into the brain. The release of such brain stimulants by hot chocolate antioxidants can be used to cure dementia; which is caused by reduced blood flow to the brain. Cocoa also could therefore have the potential to cure dementia. Drinking dark cocoa or dark chocolate daily improves man's happiness and raises man's libido and vitality.

Drinking dark chocolate or cocoa daily also strengthens men's vitality and the male sexual organ performance and therefore together with pomegranate; it is good news to wives (Song of Solomon 7:10).

REFERENCE: F.M.Steinberg, R.R.Holt, H.H.Schmitz and C.L.Keen (2002). Journal of Nutritional Biochemistry 13: 545 – 652; P. Kris-Etherton and C.L.Keen (2002). Current Opinion Lipidol13:41 – 49; www.enerhealthbotanicals.com May 2013

# CHAPTER NINE
## HEALTHY HOT SOUP DRINKS WITH NO SALT ADDED

Hot soups are needed by most people especially as warming up drinks in extremely cold weather or as pre-dinner appetisers.

1. MUSHROOM SOUP (From world class cook's recipe):
   1.1 Typical nutrient per 100g mushroom

| NUTRIENT | VALUE PER 100g |
|---|---|
| CALORIES | 175 KCAL |
| PROTEN | 9.0g |
| CARBOHYDRATE | 8.3g |
| SUGAR | 4.1g |
| FATS | 11.5g |
| SATURATES | 3.4g |
| ANTIOXIDANTS | + + |

1.1 Typical good mushroom soup ingredients : for 6 people

Mushrooms fresh from the farm: 600g of finely cut mushroom pieces (of the best local commercially farmed mushroom available: **to be safe from some unknown poisonous wild mushrooms**); olive oil, 1 small dried porcini; 2 cloves garlic peeled and finely sliced; 1 red onion peeled and finely chopped; 1 handful of thyme leaves picked up; madras curry **to replace salt** for the sake of good health (Exodus 12: 8); freshly ground black paper; 1 litre organic or vegetable stock; 1 handful fresh flat-leaf parsley leaves picked up and roughly chopped; 1 table spoon cheese; 1 lemon; and mix all thoroughly. Cook in enough but not excessive boiling water for 20 minutes and simmer for 20 minutes. Find out other interesting ways of cooking the mushroom, if necessary, as described by world class cooks for best flavours and maximum enjoyment of course.

HEALTH ALERT: Salt in the form of sodium chloride or sea salt is one of the known causes of high blood pressure as it builds up in the blood over many years of eating salty foods. It is therefore advised here to avoid table salt by replacing it with madras curry or any good curry of own choice in all the different soup recipes given in this book. You can therefore begin to treat yourself from high blood pressure by eliminating salt completely from your food and drinks or soups. Read Exodus 12: 8: '.......with bitter herbs they shall eat it'. Bitter herbs means no salt to be added!

**Health benefits of mushrooms:** Shitake or white button or any type of mushrooms such as cistini and portobello and others, all have rich content of selenium and vitamin D. Mushrooms also have phyto chemical antioxidants that reduce breast cancer and prostate cancer. Drinking hot mushroom soup especially during cold weather is not only grandmother's tale of warming us but it does have very good health benefits!

1. CHICKEN SOUP

    A typical chicken soup is made from the ingredients of chicken, carrots, onion, sweet potato, parsley, parsnip, turnips, celery, sea salt and pepper; with each vegetable ingredient bringing its own rich micronutrients into the special chicken broth of the soup.

The carrots in the chicken soup bring in a lot of vitamins including Vitamin A and carotenoids, vitamin C and other antioxidants whose health benefits have been described in the fruit juices chapter 7 in this book. Parsnips are rich in vitamin C which is also a known strong antioxidant. Turnips are rich in beta carotenes; celery is an anti-gout vegetable full of magnesium and iron that give it the anti-gout potency; and sea salt has a good balance of Na. Mg and K minerals salts to counter the bad effects of sodium salts only. Chicken contains large amounts of cysteine amino acid which helps thin out mucous in lungs of flu sufferers. Onions contain garlic which is a powerful antibody that boosts the immune system and also relieves the upper respiratory symptoms by inhibiting white neutrophils that cause the flu symptoms. Black pepper contains alkaloids and proteins and minerals with good antioxidant effect.

Chicken soup is known to cure common colds and other physical maladies during especially the colder seasons of the year. Chicken soup watery broth helps speed up recovery from a malady by rehydrating the body with the extra fluid intake from the soup. Hot chicken soup can help with nasal and throat and chest disinfection by removing bacteria from the throat, mouth and tonsils. The protein from chicken boosts energy supply and recovery processes through the enhanced protein metabolism. The advantage of chicken soup to man and family is that, almost every house hold world-wide keeps or has ready access to chicken and a variety of vegetable ingredients similar to those mentioned here.

2. BROCCOLI VEGETABLE SOUP

Broccoli in the diet of people with tumours was shown to reduce the tumour by up to 75%. Therefore broccoli prevents cancers through glucoraphanin that is converted to sulphoraphane an antibiotic that destroys *H. pylori* which is known to cause gastric cancers; also preventing breast cancers, cervical and prostate cancer.

Broccoli is rich in fibres that help the body reduce cholesterol and so preventing circulatory diseases and heart disease.

The antioxidants kaempferol, isothyanates and omega 3 fatty acids are rich nutrients of broccoli and these make the broccoli soup a good cure for allergic reactions and other body maladies.

There is also powerful antioxidant effect from broccoli soup coming from vitamin C and flavonoids which are present in the broccoli as nutrients.

Good bone strength is also promoted through the vitamin K richly present in broccoli.

Detoxification of the body by broccoli soup is promoted by glucoraphane, gluconasturtin and glucobrassicin antioxidants from broccoli and the diet is enriched with proteins and carbohydrates from broccoli. Broccoli soup also helps to give alkali pH medium to the body with the rich alkaline salts content of potassium and calcium. Typical nutrients in broccoli soup are indicated in the table 3 below.

Table 3: Typical nutrients in two types of broccoli soup per cup serving

| SOUP CATEGORY | HEALTHYCLASSIC CREAM OF BROCCOLI SOUP: LOW CALORIES CATEGORY. | CREAM OF CHEDDAR CHEESE BROCCOLI SOUP: HIGH CALORIES CATEGORY. |
|---|---|---|
| NUTRIENT | VALUE PER CUP | VALUE PER CUP |
| CALORIES | 87.8 KCAL | 430 KCAL |
| FAT | 2.8g | 31g |
| CARBOHYDRATES | 13.3g | 27g |
| PROTEIN | 5g | 14g |
| VITAMIN A | 200 IU | + + IU |
| VITAMIN C | 12mg | + + mg |
| DIETARY FIBRE | 2g | + +g |
| CALCIUM | 150mg | + +mg |
| SODIUM | 860mg | + +mg |
| CHOLESTEROL | 10mg | + +mg |
| ANTIOXIDANTS anti-cancer | + + | + + + |
| ANTIOXIDANTS anti heart disease | + + | + + + |

3. TOMATO SOUP

Tomato soup is used by many dieters as a main meal to drastically reduce weight because it is low in calories and is quick and easy to prepare from the dried tomato powder. Tomato soup also contains lycopene and the flavonoid antioxidants that fight cancers as already described in the fresh fruits and juice section of his book. The antioxidants present in the tomato soup also help to control cholesterol levels, a process that also reduces high blood pressure. Antioxidants in tomato soup are also known to help smokers recover from the toxic effects of the smoked tobacco. Tomato soup nutrients are known to promote good skin outlook through vitamin A and K; giving a glowing flawless skin. Tomato soup also has nutrients that strengthen bones, teeth, ligaments and eye sight. Typical tomato soup nutrients are shown in table 4 below.

## 4. TOMATO SOUP

Table 4: Typical nutrient tomato soup per 121g

| NUTRIENT | VALUE PER 121g |
|---|---|
| CALORIES | 121 KCAL |
| TOTAL FAT | 1g |
| SODIUM | 667mg |
| CARBOHYDRATES | 16g |
| DIETARY FIBRE | 1g |
| SUGARS | 10g |
| PROTEIN | 2g |
| VITAMIN A | 9% |
| VITAMIN C | 26% |
| CALCIUM | 2% |
| IRON | 7% |
| ANTIOXIDANTS | + + |

HEALTH ALERT: The sodium salt is too high in the ready prepared soup for people who want to reduce salt intake. Therefore it does someone good to prepare their own original vegetable tomato or broccoli soup or mushroom soup in which they can leave out the sodium salt and replace it for example; with a curry, such as madras curry.

REFERENCE: U.I. Haq, M.A. Khan, S.A. Khan and M. Ahmad (2011). Biochemical analysis of fruiting bodies of *Volvoriella vovacea* (mushroom) strain grown on six different substrates.

Soil Environment 30 (2) 146 -150. 2011.

D.A. Moreno, M.Carvaial, C.Lopez – Berenquer and C. Gareia – Viquera (2006). Chemical and biological characterisation of nutraceutical compounds of broccoli. Journal of Pharm Biomedical Anal. (2006).

B. Mahieddine, S.M. Faouzi, S. Hedjer, H. Moussa, B. Alssa and S. Mahmoud (2011). Heat treatment of effect on the technological quality of processed tomato paste. Canadian Journal on Chemical Engineering 2 (3) 27 – 40. 2011.

Jamie's Dinners by Jamie Oliver: Penguin publishers: 28 January 2010,

www.data.self.comMay2013,www.care2.com May2013;www.naturalnews.comMay2013;www.livelighter.org:May 2013.

# CHAPTER TEN
## OTHER CITRUS FRUIT JUICES
### 1. AVOCADO JUICE

Avocado juice is known to cure diabetes and Azheimers. Avocadoes have healthy omega3 fats, rich vitamin folates and vitamin E, this triple combination being very good against Azheimers. The fruit contains beta sitosterol which lowers LDL and cholesterol levels whilst raising HDL. Avocado is used as a healthy nutrient to pregnant women to supply brain developing folic acid to the foetus naturally. Avocado is known to protect against prostate and breast cancer.

1.0 Table 1.0: Typical nutrient value per 150g Avocado fruit

| NUTRIENT | VALUE PER 100G |
|---|---|
| 240 CALORIES | 184 CALORIES FROM FAT |
| FAT | 22g |
| UNSATURATED | 18% APPROX. |
| SATURATED FATS | 16% APPROX. |
| DIETARY FIBRE | 10g (40% of daily) |
| SUGARS | 1g |
| PROTEIN | 3g |
| VITAMIN A | 4% of daily |
| VITAMIN C | 25% of daily |
| IRON | 5% of daily |
| CALCIUM | 2% of daily |
| ANTIOXIDANTS | Several types of antioxidants |

Avocado is rich in several types of antioxidants that enable the fruit to give health benefits of anti-inflammation against rheumatoid arthritis and oesteoathritis. It promotes healthy adsorption of carotenoids; prevents cardiovascular diseases and accentuates blood glucose control possibly preventing diabetes and providing anti-cancer activities. Five types of the antioxidants which are also anti-inflammatory are as follows:

1. Phytosterols:(beta,.sitesterol,.stigmasterol.and coupesterol)
2. Carotenoid antioxidants: (lutein, neoxanthin, neochrome, chrysanthemaxanthin, beta cryptoxanthin, zeaxanthin, violaxanthin, B-Carotene and A-Carotene)
3. Other.antioxidants:(flavonoids,.epicatechin,.epigallocatechin, 3-0gallate, vitamin C & E, manganese, selenium and zinc)
4. Omega 3 fatty acids
5. Polyhydroxylated fatty alcohols

With all these antioxidants, avocado is indeed well packed enough to be of great health benefits for protective consumption against many diseases.

REFERENCE:

V.L. Fulgoni 3rd, M. Dreher and A.J. Davenport (2013).

Avocado consumption is associated with better diet quality and nutrient intake and lower metabolic syndrome risk in adults: results from National Health and Nutrition Examination Survey 2001 – 2008: Nutritional 12 (1). 2013.

P.F.Louis. www.naturalnews.com. April 2013.

## 2. MULBERRIES (BLACK MULBERRY) silk worm tree

**2.0 Table 2:** Health benefits from black mulberry fruit juice per 100g fruit

| NUTRIENT | VALUE PER 100G |
|---|---|
| CALORIES | ONLY 43 KCAL |
| SUGARS | 9.8g |
| PROTEIN | 1.44g |
| TOTAL FAT | 0.39g |
| CHOLESTROL | 0 |
| DIETARY FIBRE | 1.7g |
| VITAMINS | |
| FOLATE | 6ug |
| NIACIN | 0.620mg |
| PYRIDOXINE | 0.050mg |
| RIBOFLAVIN | 0.101mg |
| VITAMIN A | 25IU |
| VIT. C | 36.4mg |
| VIT. E | 0.87mg |
| VIT. K | 7.8ug |
| ELECTROLYTES: NUTRIENTS in mulberries | VALUE PER 100g |
| SODIUM | 10mg |
| POTASSIUM | 194mg |
| MINERALS | |
| CALCIUM | 39mg |
| COPPER | 60ug |
| IRON | 1.85mg |
| MAGNESIUM | 18mg |
| SELENIUM | 0.6ug |
| ZINC | 012mg |
| PHYTONUTRIENTS | |
| CAROTENE..B | 8ug |
| CAROTENE..O | 12ug |
| ZEA LUTEIN XANTHIN | 136ug |

Black mulberries are more nutritious, tasty and have greater flavour than red and white. Mulberries have low calories. They contain health promoting antioxidants in the form of anthocyanins which have anti-aging effects. These antioxidants also prevent cancers, neurological diseases, inflammation, diabetes and bacterial infections. Within the mulberries is a potent polyphenolic antioxidant called resveratrol, which protects against circulatory strokes. Mulberries have plenty of Vitamin C, amounting to 61% of daily requirement.

Other minerals and vitamin effects to health benefit have been described already in Chapters 3 to Chapter 9.

3. PURE LEMON FRUIT JUICE WITH HONEY: IN ONE CUP OF HOT BOILED WATER: AN OVERNIGHT FLU SYMPTOMS TREATMENT TONIC

Table 3: Preparation of fresh lemon juice in freshly boiled hot water and natural honey to treat flu symptoms overnight: (CAUTION: only suitable if you are not allergic to honey and lemon: also all diabetics must consult their private Doctor <u>before</u> taking this tonic)

| NUTRIENT SOURCE | VALUE IN ONE CUP OF HOT BOILED WATER: AND PRAPARATION PROCEDURE |
|---|---|
| ONE FRESH LEMON FRUIT | Cut into 2 halves: <u>squeeze out</u> all the juice <u>from one half</u> of the lemon into freshly boiled hot water in one cup full: mix well |
| NATURAL HONEY: 2 SPOONS FULL | Add 2 spoons of honey into the cup filled with freshly prepared lemon-in-hot water: mix well |
| FINAL MIXTURE OF LEMON & HONEY TONIC IN HOT WATER | Drink slowly whilst still warm from the cup |
| REPEAT OVERNIGHT AFTER 3 HOURS | Drink a freshly prepared tonic as above after 3 every hours if necessary |

The flu symptoms treatment tonic described in table3 helps to relieve severe flu symptoms when severe flu catches you at early evening time, soon after surgeries and pharmacies are closed and you just have to help yourself out overnight. It is a nutritious and very safe self-help which also gets you up the following morning well-nourished with the lemon and honey antioxidants as described in Chapter 5, table 1.2 for natural honey and in Chapter 7, table 1.1 for the lemon fruit. If you look carefully on table 1.1 Chapter 7 you will see that lemon has the highest value of vitamin C (32mg) out of the 10 fruits (except orange) and also lemon has the highest value of pyridoxine (0.8g). These high values of vitamin C and pyridoxine in lemon, when combined with the rich antioxidants of natural honey (Chapter 5 table 1.2) could well be the basis for the emergency cure effectiveness of the flu symptoms by the tonic described in table 3 here.

A PRAYER OF THANKS TO GOD: I Caleb Muzariri, thank Almighty God, our Highest Lord Jesus Christ for giving me the revelation about this anti-flu tonic, through my own Parents many years ago as a young child, now remembering to pass it on, first to my wife and then children, and now next to other people internationally; may Almighty God bless and kindly heal those who will use the anti-flu tonic.

REFERENCE: E. Tripoli, M.L. Gaurdia, S. Giammanco, D.D. Majo and M. Giammanco (2007). Citrus flavonoids: Molecular, biological activity and nutritional properties. Food Chemistry 104: (2) 466 – 479. 2007.

# CHAPTER ELEVEN

## MAKING HEALTHY FERMENTED NON ALCOHOLIC DRINKS FROM SORGHUM AND MILLET

**1.0 HEALTHY FERMENTED SORGHUM AND MILLET NON ALCOHOLIC DRINKS:** In drought prone areas and regions of the world, drought resistant crops such as sorghum and millets are very important and actually vital to the local communities. We cannot therefore underestimate the need for the technological development of the healthy processing of these foods to improve nutrition and the healthy lifestyle of their men folk. Presently the technology that exists for non-alcoholic commercial scale beverage production still presents some difficult challenges of the economics of scale, but we can still look at promoting the existing traditional technologies so that from these, innovation may eventually give rise to the scaling up; scaling up the basic traditional methods to future large scale. This is important so as to achieve the industrialization and commercialization of these cereals for the benefit of many more people in these dry regions of the world. It is not right to have a predominantly alcoholic beer brewing process for sorghum and millet for the men folk of these dry regions because alcoholic beer slowly destroys the lifestyle of men throughout the world. The purpose of this book is to promote healthy drinks and a healthy lifestyle for all men of the world. In Southern Africa for example, the tradition of brewing non-alcoholic beverages from sorghum and millet for men is nearly being made extinct by the predominantly alcoholic brewing processes for sorghum and millet for large scale commercial gain at the costly expense of men's health. In this chapter, therefore I have tried to revive the traditional brewing process of non-alcoholic beverages from sorghum and millet, so that there can at least be a re-start towards encouraging a healthy lifestyle of drinking the non-alcoholic fermented traditional drinks from sorghum and millet.

According to the Holy Bible people are saved by faith through their good works and their good deeds and therefore it is important to remind men that drinking non-alcoholic drinks not only looks good to their loving wives but also to God our Creator, our JEHOVAH. Non- alcoholic sorghum and millet drinks will also not only improve the health of men in those dry regions, but will enable men to do good works for themselves, their family and also good works for God and be saved from sins of drunkenness; with the goodness of a healthy lifestyle!

1.1 BREWING NON ALCOHOLIC HEALTHY DRINKS CALLED *BITI* OR *MASVUSVU* FROM SORGHUM OR MILLET: **This technology had almost gone extinct in Southern Africa and it is my hope and trust in God that this chapter will revive it for the health benefits of men living in the dry regions of Southern Africa where only sorghum and millet are predominant sources of daily food.**

1.2 PREPARING SORGHUM OR MILLET FOR NON ALCOHOLIC DRINK PRODUCTION:

The grain is firstly put through the usual grinding process to produce a fine mealy mill dry powder at the local grinding mill. The ground mealy mill is then ready to be used for making both staple food and the healthy non-alcoholic drink.

1.3 BOILING THE CLEAN BREWING WATER TO MAKE A SWEET HEALTHY *BITI* OR *MASVUSVU*

For maximum benefit and for the economics of brewing the drink once every two weeks; and storing enough to be consumed over several days once it is decided to brew the sweet beverage, a minimum of 20 litres of the brewing water should be used each time so as to save on cooking coals or firewood or electricity.

Place 20 litres of the brewing water into a suitably prepared large 20 litre clay pot or hygienically tested safe, properly manufactured stainless steel 20 litre kitchen pot or small scale stainless steel brewing pot. Bring the 20 litres of water to boil on a suitable fire.

## 1.4 THE BREWING OF SWEET NON ALCOHOLIC *BITI* OR *MASVUSVU*

As soon as the 20 litres of water comes to boiling point, quickly add 200 grams or 2 cups full of fine ground mealy mill of sorghum grain or millet grain, stirring gently all round within the clay pot with a long enough wooden stirrer. Keep the mealy mill brew evenly distributed and dispersed throughout the whole boiling water. Reduce heat but continue cooking the liquid brew for up to 3 hours, remembering to stir it regularly. About 2.5 hours into the brewing cooking process, just before you start cooling the brew, add 20 very clean fresh green leaves of the sweet fruit-producing *muhacha* tree (*muhacha* tree leaves is a good traditional alternative to what hops do to alcohol beer brewing!). If you cannot find *muhacha* tree leaves, use an equivalent number of sweet *muzhanje* tree fresh green leaves. Stir the sweet fruit tree green leaves gently throughout your brew. After 3 hours of cooking and mixing the non- alcoholic healthy sweet drink brew, put out the cooking fire or heat to allow the 20 litre brew to slowly cool down. Sweeten the cooling brew by adding *hacha* fruit juice prepared by crushing the *hacha* fruit and extracting the *hacha* fruit juice with hot boiled water or use similar suitable fruit juice as sweetening juice at the end of the 3 hours. Allow the whole 20 litre brew to continue fermenting in a cool room with plenty of fresh air for up to 24 hours. The formation of white bubbling foam on top of your new sweet beverage indicates that it is getting ready as a good drink. Diabetics must not add any sugar to the beverage; and generally for everyone, to prevent long term diabetics problems for every healthy person, use sweet fresh fruit juices as sweeteners of your drink and do not use sugar. When it tastes ready; you can add to taste if you like, natural honey or some brown sugar and then dispense your sweet brew into several smaller containers for long term storage in the refrigerator or very cool room. Enjoy the healthy drink up to several days and avoid drinking alcoholic beer so as to get used to a new healthy lifestyle of healthy, fruity tasty drinks with plenty of antioxidants and vitamins (table 1.2). These antioxidants in sorghum or millet prevent many diseases whilst making the men stronger and healthier and much happier saving a lot of money that would be wasted in buying the very destructive alcoholic beers of all sorts!. May God bless you the new non-alcoholic drinker and move on to a new healthy lifestyle with your happy family!

Table 1.2 here shows the potential health benefits of a typical sorghum and a millet liquid extract: (Modified from C.C Muzariri: 2008: pp 34 and pp 39: M.Phil Thesis: University of Manchester, School of Chemical Engineering and Analytical Science)

| NUTRIENTS FROM SORGHUM | COMPOSITON % |
|---|---|
| ZEAXANTHIN | 36.3 |
| LUTEIN | 28.6 |
| *B*- CAROTENE | 10.4 |
| **PHENOLIC COMPOUNDS WITH HEALTH BENEFITS IN BOTH SORGHUM AND MILLET** | |
| HYDROXYBENZOIC ACIDS | PRESENCE IN SORGHUM OR MILLET |
| GALLIC ACID | Present in sorghum and millet |
| PROTOCATECHUIC | Present in sorghum and millet |
| *p*-HYDROXYBENZOIC ACID | Present in sorghum and millet |
| GENTISIC | Present in sorghum and millet |
| SALICYLIC | In sorghum only |
| SYRINGIC | Present in sorghum and millet |
| HYDROXYCINNAMIC ACIDS | |
| FERULLIC | Present in sorghum and millet |
| CAFFEIC | Present in sorghum and millet |
| *p*-COUMARIC | Present in sorghum and millet |
| CINNAMIC | Present in sorghum and millet |
| SINAPIC | Present in sorghum and millet |

These above listed antioxidants in sorghum and millets have also been discussed from fruits in Chapter 7 in this book; about their effectiveness against cancers, prostate cancer, against diabetes, against high blood pressure. Therefore men (and their wives too!) drinking non-alcoholic tasty drinks brewed from sorghum and millet will be protected from many diseases as well as finally freeing themselves from the bad unhealthy trappings of drinking all sorts of alcoholic beers! All women in the dry regions of the world where sorghums and millets are being predominantly used to brew only alcoholic beers must move on to help out their men by starting to brew tasty non-alcoholic beverages from sorghum and millet because these are healthy for their men and for the women themselves also.

May God bless all the men and women of the sorghum and millet regions of the world with new healthy non-alcoholic drinks and new healthy recipes from the sorghum and millet cereal processed grains.

## 1.5 POTENTIAL BIOTECHNOLOGICAL IMPROVEMENT OF *BITI* AND *MASVUSVU* BY FINDING A SUITABLE PROBIOTIC MICRORGANISM THAT PRODUCES BY FERMENTAION SWEETENING FRUCTOSE WITHIN THE *BITI*; SIMILAR TO COMMERCIAL LACTOBACTER USED IN YOGURTS:

Adding fruit juices to the final brewed *Biti* or *Masvusvu* may not be an economic way to make the best beverage out of sorghum and millet if for example sweet wild fruits or orchard fruits are not available for the community. Recently some researchers have shown that sweet fructose is produced from the carbohydrate inulin through a microbial fermentation (Lima et al). An innovative *Biti* and *Msvusvu* fermentation is required to produce sweet fructose from within the *Biti* fermentation glucose-rich beverage. A microorganism that converts sugars to sweet fructose within the *Biti* beverage would be a major breakthrough for a much richer probiotic *Masvusvu* beverage which could also be commercialised to provide more communities with a healthy and tasty non-alcoholic beverage with very healthy nutrients. Adding citric acid to the brewed *Biti or Masvusvu* can also improve the flavour and storage quality of the non-alcoholic sorghum or millet beverages

REFERENCE:

Caleb Muzariri (2009). Debranning milling processes of wheat and sorghum. M.Phil Thesis. School of Chemical Engineering and Analytical Sciences: University of Manchester

Caleb C Muzariri (1994). Citric Acid. A Review. In: Food Science and Technology: Challenges for Africa towards the year 2000. Edit. L. Marovatsanga and J.N. Taylor. ISBN 0-908507.

Fructose: A Biotechnology Asset: D. D. Lima, P. Fernandes, D.S. Nascimento, R. de Cassia, F. Ribeiro and S. A. de Assis: Food Technology Biotechnology 49 (4): 424-434 (2011).

# CHAPTER TWELVE

## MAKING HEALTHY FERMENTED FRUIT AND MILK PRODUCTS: THE POTENTIAL HEALTH BENEFITS OF FERMENTED NON ALCOHOLIC FRUIT YOGURTS: YOGURTS FROM DIFFERENT FRUITS

Fermented yogurt was started during the early Biblical times by Abraham as he prepared to meet the three angels sent to bless him by Almighty God just before the conception of his beloved son Isaac by his wife Sarah at the time of Biblical Genesis (Genesis verses). We should therefore regard yogurt as one of the special foods directly blessed for our own good by almighty God; including the pomegranate fruit which we can use to make fruit favoured yogurt.

1. MAKING YOGURT BY MILK FERMENTATION

Milk if unpasteurised and left at room temperature naturally ferments; and this is what Abraham must have observed on how to make cheese in Biblical Genesis time.

### 1.1 YOGURT MAKING INGREDIENTS AND DOMESTIC TECHNOLOGY: METHOD 1:

I. Use 2.5 litres of whole milk, raw or pasteurized; cow or goat milk.
II. Milk Lactic acid bacteria Starter Culture: Use Commercial Starter reading carefully package instructions; OR Use 2 tablespoons full of your favourite yogurt line culture; have a Thermometer ready; Have your yogurt maker oven (or commercial incubator ready at 43 °C; OR a Cooler Box with water at 43 °C ready.

III. THE YOGURT MAKING PROCEDURE:
1. Heat the milk up to 43 °C checking temperature with the thermometer.
2. Cool down the milk to 43 °C if the temperature overshot above 43 °C.
3. Add starter culture of the yogurt and stir in thoroughly into the milk.
4. Dispense the milk into your glass jars with screw cups covers and place the milk-filled glass jars into the oven at 43 °C; making sure that your oven light is on to keep the temperature at 43 °C; OR Use industrial incubator set at 43 °C.
5. Keep the milk in the jars at 43 °C for 4 hours to 10 hours; 4 hours produces mild yogurt; 10 hours produces the mature tangy yogurt.
6. UNCONVENTIONAL METHOD OF MAKING YOGURT: If your oven cannot keep temperature constant at 43 °C, use a Cooler Box with water at 43 °C; keeping thermometer ready in the box; topping up with hot water into the box after some hours when it drops below 43 °C. Make sure you keep temperature around 43 °C though out for the 4 to 10 hours; so as to harvest a good yogurt.
7. To make a thicker yogurt, heat the milk up to 82 °C and then let it cool down to 43 °C before adding starter culture. Then add fruit, honey or other flavours.
8. Make your thick fruit or flavoured yogurt at 43 °C.

9. PLACES TO BUY YOGURT MAKING STARTER CULTURES: some of them are as follows: 1. Stay

Cultured.com 2. Cheese-Yogurt-Making.com. 3. Several other good sources of edible probiotic starter cultures online.

With this domestic technology it is therefore possible to make your own fermented yogurts to personal satisfaction and family satisfaction. May God bless you as you make these healthy foods for yourselves and we all must always pray to thank God for the good food and drinks that He gives us.

## 1.2 MAKING LACTOSE-FREE YOGURT AND DOMESTIC TECHNOLOGY: METHOD 2:

1. Use 4 cups of milk; for best yogurt use milk from grass fed cows.
2. STERILISE your kitchen yogurt making equipment to get good quality yogurt.
3. Pour the 4 cups of milk in a heavy bottom pot or pan and let it heat up to medium temperature, stirring the milk so that it does not burn on to the pot.
4. Heat up to 82 °C using THERMOMETER to check the temperature or see bubbles forming on the edges of the pot or pan: heating up to 82 °C until bubbles start forming kills unwanted bacteria so that you can add your starter into pasteurized milk.
5. Cool to room temperature your pasteurized milk.
6. ADD THE STARTER CULTURE after reading carefully the commercial instructions on the commercial supplier's starter bottle. OR If using leftover yogurt; prepare about ½ cup of the cooled milk mixed with ¼ cup of leftover yogurt. Mix in the ½ cup pasteurized milk & ¼ cup leftover ALL into the rest of the cooked pasteurized milk. Add fruit or other flavour at this stage and mix thoroughly.

7. Dispense the cultured cooked milk into your glass jars as usual.
8. Cover the glass jars with plastic wrap and place them in the oven with the light open; at 43 °C; checking temperature with THERMOMETER.
9. Let the milk ferment for 24 hours so as to get rid of all LACTOSE TO MAKE THE LACTOSE-FREE YOGURT
10. THE LACTOSE-FREE YOGURT is ready after 24 hours fermentation in the oven at 43 °C.
11. Store your yogurt jars in the refrigerator, ready to enjoy your yogurt.

1.3 HEALTH BENEFITS OF YOGURTS: Yogurt brings into the stomach health beneficial probiotics which reverse some diseases whilst improving immunity; bowel health and overall good health. The fruit juice-treated yogurt also carries with it all the good antioxidants of the fruit as described for each type of fruit in Chapter 7. Therefore from table 1.2 in Chapter 7 you can actually pick and choose which best fruit-flavoured yogurt to make for yourself so as to build up specific antioxidants that you personally need at any particular time. The probiotics in the yogurt also naturally produce more vitamins and nutrients, adding to more antioxidants towards your health benefits. Finally an important Biblical quote: "Butter and honey shall He eat............" (Isaiah 7: 15).

REFERENCE: O. Adolfsson, S.N. Meydani and R. Russell (2004). Yogurt and gut function 1'2. 2004.American Society for Clinical Nutrition.

P. Bourdioux and P. Pochart (1988). Nutritional and health benefits of yogurt. World Rev. Nutr. Diet (1988) 56: 217 – 258.

wholehealthsource.blogspot.co.uk: S. Guyenet: 16 March 2008;

Paleodietlifestyle.com/homemade-yogurt: May 2013.

## CHAPTER THIRTEEN
## HEALTHY ENDURANCE TRAINING AND MAXIMUM PREPARATION TO BE A TOP WORLD CLASS ATHLETE OR SPORTSMAN

1.0 PRACTICE AND PRACTICE AND PRACTICE IN YOUR FAVOURITE SPORTS SPECIALITY FROM THE EARLIEST AGE POSSIBLE AND BE HIGHLY COMPETITIVE AT ALL LEVELS OF DEVELOPMENT:

It is very important to be really interested in your chosen field of sports and plan to excel in it. If it is football at your boys school of 400 boys, all totally motivated school boys; you must know that the school coach will only need to pick up at the most only 24 excellent boys in football for the school first and second teams. You must therefore skilfully brace yourself for intense competition with the other 399 school boys to make it into the top 11 great footballers of the school of the school's first team. That requires good self-discipline, obedience to your parents and to your teachers so that you have good all round support. A good Christian young man will have a good habit of being obedient to Almighty God by reading the Bible and praying to our Lord Jesus Christ for spiritual guidance especially as the competition for the top 11 best footballers in the local City gets much more intense than it would have been at school. Treat yourself to a healthy lifestyle of avoiding health damaging alcoholic drinks or drugs and smoking and be a leader even to your peers leading them by good lifestyle example of drinking only healthy non-alcholic drinks as you practice hard daily for your favourite sports. And be humbly proud of your thriving sportsmanship so that even your friends will see how good it is to be successful without using unhealthy substances. The more you practice hard on your football or athletics more often by yourself, often in your own privacy, the greater the chances of making it to the top because when you then after meet others at the common training football pitch or athletics track, you will already be miles ahead with your own private endurance training. That makes you that special for a good start! Learn the scientific skills, biochemistry and physiology sports physical training; including the health aspects that is needed in your own sports speciality by taking the relevant sports option in your school's daily activities; but not neglecting other life skills courses.

## 1.1 MY OWN ATHLETICS TRAINING AS AN EXAMPLE:

I remember getting seriously into 100 meters and 200 meters training at the early age of seven years old. From that time going to school, coming from school and at school sports events, I always competitively raced very fast either with friend or brother. Build yourself up gradually but strongly plan to be the best among the best. A future world 100 meters athletics champion does not settle for second best at any level, from junior school, secondary school, throughout College years. If there is going to be a 100 meter new world record holder; there is only going to be one such champion and if you decide it is going to be you; young man (or woman so as to also advise women athletes) plan for it <u>every day.</u> Every day of training; because you only make it to world record on that very special one day after preparing yourself for the challenge, daily, over many years. This is how I made it to my own 'unofficial' 100 meter world record. I did not just rise that morning to go and race my friends at the track; I strongly trained daily at every level of my youth development from boys' age, through teens and up to early stages as a young man at 18 years old; the very time I made it for that great achievement. If it can be afforded, have your own private gym which has appropriate muscles development equipment. Get a good coach to advise you from an early age; and in modern athletics there are many good coaches who can help you for free. The best coach you can have is one who accepts Lord Jesus Christ as our Saviour because they are most likely to complement your alcohol-free and drugs-free, smoking-free lifestyle and to help you pray to God; but by God's own Grace some many coaches who do not go to church also have the good habits of alcohol-free and drugs-free lifestyle and if you get such a coach; thank God but try to teach them your own best skill; and that is how to pray to God! our Lord Jesus Christ. Teach also your training team friends to pray to God; and never be swayed by friends from praying to God especially the more you succeed; stand firm and be the leader of good friends and refuse to be led by bad habit friends; especially the more you succeed, thank God for your flourishing talents. Give tithes to your local Christian church to get more blessings from God as you succeed more and more; as you train harder towards your best athletics performance ever!

Eat healthy foods and avoid junk foods; plenty of fresh fruits from young age; drink fresh fruit drinks and milk at the early young age as you daily practice the highest speed of sprinting you can achieve each day. Choose the best healthy drinks from those that have been fully described for you in this book. In addition, as a young Christian, trust our Lord Jesus Christ by your daily prayers and Bible reading; you will enjoy God's blessings by the greatest achievement God will enable you.

**1.2** HOW TO TRAIN ON SPEED AS FUTURE NEW WORLD RECORD 100 METER COMPETITOR:

It is vital that a 100 meter sprinter trains on skilful and disciplined starting at the starting block, timing, achieving the best speed, powering forward, leading with strength, muscular flexibility, good coordination and eliminating fatigue by strong and consistent endurance training.

> a. **Skilful and disciplined starting at the starting block**:

This requires a high degree of self-discipline and alertness to listen and react to the starter pistol sound, timing to start off the starting block, avoiding either slow start or faulty starts. You need to thoroughly train yourself so to regularize a high level of faultless starting off as this decides your very future championship. Insist that your coach facilitates training regularly on the best explosive start off, practicing daily and every week, demand the best.

> b. **Timing your sprint:**

Timing your sprint means timing how fast and how strongly you are going to surge ahead of any other competitor in your hits or final race. It simply means if it is at the hits, aim to be the first to cross the finish line; and at the final, aim to be the champion to first cross the finishing line and celebrate. Be strong and tough and never accept second best in your timing. To achieve strong timing, every 100 meter champion sprinter (male or female) has to train for strong leg and body muscle development at the gym, weights lifting or pulling weights by your waist and exercising your legs correctly. Know the current world record and daily aim to move as close to it as possible asking your coach to continuously monitor your timing progressions every week and every month throughout the whole year.

> c. **Achieving the best speed and powering forward:**

This means be determined and self-motivated to win against the strongest of your competitors at any time and any at event. Be aware of the biggest threat and watch them with the eye of an eagle to make sure you thwart their own speed as you power forward for a vital win and if necessary set a new record simply because you must be the winner in that race! This means you must be highly competitive to be the best. This is where God given sheer talent supported by self-disciplined training also plays a very big part. For a good Christian young athlete, the power of prayer and tithing brings in that extra motivation for which, thanks giving to our living God Lord Jesus Christ, brings more blessings.

    d. **Leading strength, muscular flexibility, good coordination and eliminating fatigue:**

The above statement looks loaded; but it simply means if you are to be the winner <u>learn to keep your lead in any sprint race and do not give up before the finishing line.</u> When you have started off well at the starting block, power forward all the time until you be the first to cross the finishing line. To achieve this you will have skilfully trained yourself not to have muscle crumbs midst the sprint, flexing your muscles strongly to keep you ahead of the other tough competitor just behind you (threatening to beat you to it if you lose coordination and get fatigued before the finishing line!). Keep your strong muscle coordination until after you have crossed the finishing line. This is where pre-final thorough practice, gym training and endurance training pays you off at the 'world championship' as you clock your new world record or your local national record for a start. Of course all this becomes real on that day because you will have had healthy drinks and healthy foods throughout your training over the many years and having a healthy life style; always remembering to pray to God thanking Him for enabling you to achieve the greatest.

# CHAPTER FOURTEEN
## HOW TO EXERCISE AND KEEP FIT AS A MAN AT WORK DAILY

1. THE SELF DESCIPLINE AND HUMBLENESS OF PRAYER AND FASTING: PRAYER AND FASTING FOR EXAMPLE FOR ONE DAY A WEEK TO THANK GOD FOR EVERTHING HE IS ENABLING US TO DO:
   The Holy Bible says fast privately and pray so that only God our Lord Jesus Christ knows that you are fasting and praying. This is good Christian self-discipline to thank God in a quiet and humble way for the great things He enables us to do. Choose your own day of fasting per week from early in the morning to 16.00pm, without taking any food, although depending on your own self health assessment, you may or may not drink water during the fasting. Fasting with no food intake is a healthy spiritual exercise because the body is resting the digestive processes in the stomach during the fasting. Immediately after fasting take in fluids gradually as you prepare the stomach for food digestion and take the food on top of the fluids first taken in, to prevent constipation. As usual of course drink your water requirement to the more than 2 litres per day after the fasting. The prayer and fasting shows our obedience to God and humbling ourselves in thanks to our God who so loved us that He gave us His only begotten Son, our Lord Jesus Christ (1 John 4: 9); and it is a good exercise of showing our trust in God.
2. TITHING TO YOUR CHURCH (WHETHER ANGLICAN, CATHOLIC, METHODIST OR FIFMI OR ANY OTHER) TO THANK GOD BY GIVING TO GOD'S HOUSE ONLY A 10$^{TH}$ OF WHAT GOD HAS GIVEN YOU IN TOTAL EARNIGS, SO THAT HE BLESSES YOU WITH MORE STRENGTH TO

WORK AND MORE PROSPERITY AND PROTECTS YOU FROM THE DEVIL (DEVOURER):

Tithing keeps you fit spiritually as an obedient child of God knowing that it is God who gives us our weekly and monthly earnings by His Grace of enabling us to work (Malachi 3: 10). Tithing enables you to put your own contribution into the work of God that your church is doing and to help build or service your local church. Do not think you are giving it to persons in the church, but you are giving it to God so as to earn your blessing (Malachi 3: 10-11) by building your own particular church as you contribute in the day to day running costs of your local church such as paying for heating bills, water bills and general up keep of the church building, so that it is always there for your local group prayers. Therefore the TITHE is God's money to make Him look after you, to protect you and to bless you more (Malachi 3: 8, 10). When you have given your tithe to your local church, you will see how free this makes you and how happy it makes you. Tithing also makes you prosperous and feel great content in your exercises knowing that you have obeyed God our Father, our living God Jesus Christ. God will look after you and will strengthen you and prosper you as you exercise and do your work. Give your wife to go with the TITHE money for you to your local church so that you make her know and respect what you are doing for the house of God. Then go to the gym for exercises if you like and she will love you more for being a good man of God. My own parents taught me tithing and giving when I was a young school boy, but then I did not quite understand what it really means in the building of the house of God, directly or indirectly. I thank God for I now know how it gives me more blessings from God. It is the best spiritual exercise to one's own salvation and blessings and it also blesses the others that your tithes help. Tithing makes you and I prosper and stronger through God's own loving power. Abraham obeyed God with the tithing and was blessed abundantly (Genesis 12); including his children from generation to generation and forever as God promised him (Genesis 12).

SOME POSSIBLE USES OF TITHES IN YOUR LOCAL CHURCH: Besides paying for daily running costs, the tithes that you and others pay monthly or weekly (according to your own specific dates of pay) to your own local church whether Anglican church, Catholic, Methodist church, FIFMI church, or Other church will be used responsibly by your own church Pastor for example to host troubled children in your local community. The tithes for example will enable children to be taught by your Pastor about responsible citizenship and salvation by our Lord Jesus CHRIST our JEHOVAH and how to become leading Christian citizens of tomorrow. As such God will bless you richly for such good causes involving development of children (and all others in need) through your own tithes individually at your own local church (Malachi 3). That is a very healthy lifestyle for every Christian man to do and you and your family will be blessed by God in His own great way.

3. PHYSICAL EXERCISES WITHOUT HAVING TO GO TO THE GYM

There are many ways to keep yourself very fit without having to spend time and money going to the gym; although if you can afford the time and money, go to the gym, it is also good. There are now so many in-own-home exercising video instructions available on the market that can take you through personal routines of exercises in your own house. Without those video instructions you can also achieve the best exercise by selecting the most free 30 minutes of your daily time allocation after work to do your own exercise routines. The best is to start by an outdoor run and walk run and walk exercise for 2 to 5 miles. The run and walk exercise means you are really doing what you like to avoid exhausting yourself. You can run hard for 200 hundred meters for example if you are running uphill and the slowdown to walk for about 300 meters, building up more fresh air into your lungs; then run for example downhill for 400 meters and then walking uphill for 800 meters or more as you like until you finish 30 minutes of your daily exercise. If you run and walk for only 15 minutes outside; you can finish the remainder 15 minutes indoors, doing healthy press ups in your own privacy. For example you can do press ups against the wall in your bathroom; pressing your two hands whilst standing about a meter away from the wall then pressing whole body weight against the wall, counting up to 150 press ups each time; then next exercise your legs by a 150 runs on the same spot in your private exercise room. The against-the-wall press ups strengthen your arms as if you are actually doing weight lifting in the gym; your arms and legs get stronger also because, as you press your arms against the wall you are also pressing on your legs to keep you firmly up from going down. That type of press up is not strenuous to your knees and it gives you a win win exercise for both arms and legs and keeps you strong and fit as those who lift weights at the gym! If you have done your exercise late at night, remember to read your Bible verses and praying to God after your shower or bath before going to bed.

4. PHYSICAL EXERCISE AT THE GYM WHEN YOU CAN AFFORD THE TIME AND COST:

Training exercises at the gym involves the use of treadmills, to run on the treadmill or to walk on the treadmill indoors. This becomes handy when the weather outside does not allow for running outside. Lifting weights at the gym also is part of the exercise routines for which you pay your money to make use of the equipment. A typical gym also has arm flexing equipment where you use your arms to turn a treadmill as you either walk or run on that self-propelled tread mill. If your house has sufficient space, most of the machines found at the gym can also be affordable to buy and put them in your own gym at home for the benefit of you and your family. That home indoor gym, in my view, is the best way to keep fit, because you can combine it flexibly with your own outdoor exercises. In the long run the cost of own equipment at home will over some time save a lot of more money that you would have paid for at a company's owned gym.

5. PHYSIOLOGICAL AND BIOCHEMICAL HEALTH BENEFITS OF EXERCISING OR DOING SPORTS

Warburton et al (2006) discussed the evidence available on the health benefits of physical exercises or activities by individuals. They identified from several medical publications that there is irrefutable evidence that exercising pays off with good health benefits; they found evidence of the effectiveness of regular exercises in the primary and secondary prevention several chronic diseases; for example, cardiovascular, diabetes, cancer, hypertension, obesity, depressions, osteoporosis and premature necrosis. They were able to confirm that a linear relationship exists between increasing exercises and improved health status and well-being of individuals. On the other extreme end those living a sedentary passive lifestyle were much more afflicted by chronic diseases and premature necrosis. The medical research results are an important eye opener to all men to keep fit by continuously exercising and drinking plenty of water and other healthy drinks to ensure a strong well-being.

Fathers must also make sure their children keep exercising enough. M.S. Sothern et al (1998) observed that children who regularly exercised were free from chronic disease, unlike those who were not exercising. Those children not exercising were found to be more prone to chronic diseases. Children and adolescents who were vulnerable to diseases such as diabetes but exercised adequately were better off health-wise. Increased activities by the children also biochemically and physiologically showed health benefits on increased low density protein and decreased high density protein, showing healthy cardiovascular systems, protection from cancers and diabetes.

## 5.1 INDOOR SPORTS EXERCISES AND OTHER OUTDOOR SPORTS

Table tennis is one of the very good indoor sports that can keep people busy running up and down for hours within the indoors. Those men folk with a spare room (after all your children have grown up and gone away to their own purchased houses) can buy themselves the affordable table and kit for table tennis. With that table tennis kit men folk can start playing table tennis with their wives instead of sitting down too much watching the television. Playing table tennis with wife can bring back the old romance to spice up a healthy lifestyle for both husband and wife. It makes the two get closer once more together rekindling the early young days of blissful romance that had long disappeared with the yelling arrival of child after child after child! If Lord Jesus Christ our living God has blessed us with our children who after growing up, all later go away to their own spouses; we should thank God and order ourselves games to play with our spouses.

In the Holy Bible, it is written Abraham continued to play with his wife Sarah when both were beyond 100 years old!

Another indoor sports for good exercise is squash, but squash needs much larger room than tennis and therefore it is a no no in your own house; but it can be possible somewhere in your own back garden. The same applies to lawn tennis; it is possible somewhere in your back garden where you can show your grandchildren that you are a very sporty granddad who whips up the tennis ball!

## 5.2 OTHER OUTDOOR SPORTS

Golf is a sports of long walks if you like long walks and hitting the small hard ball. It needs good weather and a good club; but it could make you neglect your old spouse by taking you too much out with the lads. So is cricket, which takes literally the whole day to get a final result when your spouse is patiently waiting?

Whatever you do exercise and exercise; and always pray to our Lord Jesus Christ our living God for giving us joy and salvation and all the blessings of healthy foods and a healthy lifestyle and many other good things of life. Always give tithes to your local church and that way, you will be doing great works of keeping supplied and serviced with electricity and water, God's temple at your local church (Malachi 3:10-11).

REFERENCES: Canadian Medical Association Journal: 14 March 2006: 174: 747 – 749: D.E.R. Warburton, C.W. Nicol and S.S.D. Bredin: Health benefits of physical activity: the evidence.

European Journal of Paedriatics 158: 271 – 274: M.S. Sothern, M. Loftin, R.M. Suskind, J.N. Udall and U.B. Blecker: The health benefits of physical activity in children and adolescents: implications for chronic disease prevention.

Drew Harrison and Tom Comyns (2002 – 2013): Biomechanics of the Sprint Start; University of Limerick: Ireland

## MY DAILY INSPIRATION

I believe and thank God that we were all created by God through Adam and Eve (Psalm 71: 6)

I believe that I am blessed with an inheritance as per promise by God to Abraham, Isaac and Jacob (Genesis 12)

I believe that my salvation comes from our heavenly Father, God, His Son who is also our living God, Jesus Christ and the Holy Spirit our Comforter; all the above comprising the Holy Trinity. Amen

THANKING GOD: It took me many months, up to several years, of pondering and thinking how to write this book and I continued to pray to God, not for the book, but for other blessings; and suddenly our living God, our Highest Lord Jesus Christ opened up my mind and gave me a vision of how the book should look like. As soon as I started writing it, I could not stop for a day without writing something. I thank our living God Jesus Christ, our JEHOVAH for giving me the vision and a healthy life style of prayers to Him our only God to be able to finally write this book. Galatians 1: 3. Psalm 91:4.

**PRAYER:** May our Highest Lord Jesus Christ our living JEHOVAH, our only Creator God, and His Holy Spirit bless the writer, publisher and all readers of this book. Amen

**PERSONAL THANKS:** My special thanks for good technical assistance in typesetting this book; to my daughters, Farirai Victoria, Claire Rutendo and Christina Kiri; thanks to my son Joel for his prayers for me, and their mainini Fiona Nyaradzo for encouragement and prayers, and their mother Florety Ndomupeyi for good food as I wrote this book and for encouraging our children family prayers; to my sisters; Mosti, Ennie, Angela and Agatha: Penina, Violet, Margareth, Musa, Muchaneta, Keresiya and Esnathi; Margie, Josephine and Rumbi; Martha and Miriam for prayers for me and for encouragement.

## ABOUT THE AUTHOR

Caleb Chikomba Muzariri is presently a book writer and publisher for books of Science for Christians and People of Faith (SCPF). Caleb graduated from the University of Sussex with a B.Sc. Honours degree in Biochemistry in 1977. Caleb then proceeded to the then University of Rhodesia from 1978 to 1980 training many MBCHB first and second year medical students in Biochemistry laboratory practical experiments, including setting up and marking Biochemistry and Physiology examination practical experiments for the MBCHB students; whilst Caleb also worked on his Master of Philosophy thesis in Biochemistry. From 1980, as the University of Rhodesia was renamed the University of Zimbabwe, Caleb continued his work with the new University of Zimbabwe on part-time basis as Caleb joined the Harare Polytechnic as full time Lecturer-in Charge of Science Technology from 1980 to 1985. In 1985 Caleb was promoted to full time Head of Science Technology at Harare Polytechnic and Chairman of the National Science Examinations Committee of Polytechnics and Technical Colleges in Zimbabwe. Caleb did lead the training of hundreds of science industrial laboratory technicians from his Department at Harare Polytechnic and other national Colleges. Caleb did also lead the Department to grow into a new School of Science Technology that introduced for the first time in that country; Honours Degrees in Applied Sciences as follows: Honours Degree in Applied Biology and Biochemistry; Honours Degree in Applied Chemistry and Chemical Technology; Honours Degree in Applied Physics and Mathematics. These new Honours Degrees were all transferred to the new National University of Science Technology in 1989 and Caleb went back full time to the University of Zimbabwe in December 1989 as full time Lecturer in Biochemistry up to 1999. From 2000 to 2003 Caleb joined the University of the Free State, Bloemfontein, South Africa as a Research Collaborator and Partner on a WARFSA project dealing with studies on effluent water pollution control from the pulp and paper industries using fungal and bacterial based technology. Whilst briefly back from South Africa; in 2003 to 2004 Caleb linked up with the School of Chemical Engineering and Analytical Science at the then world class UMIST in Manchester, UK; joining the UMIST in 2004 as Part time Teaching Assistant whilst working on a PhD thesis. In 2005 the UMIST was merged by politicians with the then University of Manchester to become the new University of Manchester. Caleb became Tutor of Science students in the special MAP programme of the University of Manchester and teaching Assistant to M.Sc students up to the year 2008 as Caleb wrote an M. Phil thesis when funds ran out far too short with no sponsor available to complete the PhD projects.

In addition to the above Caleb also did an HND in Analytical Biochemistry and Pharmacology at the then Brighton Polytechnic (now University of Brighton), Sussex, in association with Brighton Technical College in 1974. Recently Caleb also did part-time NVQ (UK) Level 2 in 2009 and NVQ Level 3 in 2011 both in Health, People's Welfare and Social Care. This enables Caleb to teach students in Health and Social Care or student Nutritionists for which this book is also recommended.

Caleb has always worked as a Christian Lecturer throughout his work.

TESTIMONY: I believe in God's power in His Mighty Science of Creation of people, creation of all living things and the universe through Jesus Christ our Highest Lord whom He sent here on earth to come and redeem us all (1 John 4: 9). Let us all praise our Mighty Lord Jesus Christ our living JEHOVAH our only God in whom we trust (Psalm 150).

RECOMMENDED FURTHER READINGS FOR MEN OF INTEGRITY TO KNOW MORE ABOUT GOD'S LOVE AND POWER:

1. The Holy Bible from Genesis to Revelation.
2. A Wise Man, A Real Man, A Man of Integrity: by Archbishop Professor Ezekial Guti: ISBN: 9781779120694: EGEA Publ.

# INDEX

## A
A.-type proanthocyanidins 35
Abimelech 9
Abraham 3, 9, 16, 18, 32, 60, 89
Acetic acid 32
Alcohol-free 84
Almighty God 3, 8, 33
Alminium 14
Amino acids 10, 32
amoeba 13
anaemia 35
Anglican church 91
Anthocyanins 41, 51
anti -colon cancer 37
Anti-aging 37, 38, 44, 45, 51, 60, 70
anti-athritis 44, 67
Anti-Azheimer's 39, 48
antibacterial 33, 35
antibreast.cancer.37, 38, 50
anti-cancer 19 35, 37, 40, 43, 49
Anticommon.cold38
Anti-flu tonic 71, 72
antigingivitis 38, 40
Anti-HIV 46
Anti-inflammatory 48, 67
anti-oxidant 19, 37, 41, 43, 47, 56, 58, 59, 60, 61, 65, 66, 67, 68, 71, 72
Anti-prosttate.cancer 37, 45, 46, 50, 77
antiviral 20
Apple 43, 50
Ark 8
Aspirin like effects 60
Athletics.11.,22,47
Athlete's lifestyle 43

Auto-feed machine 54
Avocado 68

## B
bacteria 14
bacteria-free 12
bacteriostatic
Banana fruit 43, 44, 45
Baptism 7
Baptism immersion 7
Baptism water 7
baptized in water 7
Bees 33
Beneficialprobiotics 81
beta carotene 19, 37, 38, 45, 50, 54
bicarbonates 15
biotin 18
Biti 74, 75
black tea 20
blessings 89
blood glucose control 67
blood platelets 19
blood pressures (bps) 10, 11
blood stream 10
Blue grapes 37, 38
Blueberries39 Betaine 39
body cells 7, 19
borates 15
born again believer 7
born again Christian 7
bottled water 10
bowel cancer 17
Brain stimulus 44, 61
Broccoli soup 64, 65
Bromelain 49
butter 17

## C
cancers 3, 18, 20

calcium 15, 19, 28, 30
Caleb 32
calories 57, 58, 66, 69
carbohydrates 10
carbon.block cartridge 12
cardiovascular system improvement 36, 37, 47
catechin 20
Catholic church 91
centrifugal 33
Cherries 39
chicken soup 64
chlorine 12, 15
chocolate 57
cholera *14*
cholesterol 20, 28, 29, 57
Christian 7
Christian parents 26
chromium 19, 37
Citric acid 32
clean athlete 27
cocoa 56, 61
cocoanut shell 15
coenzyme Q10 19
colloidal liquid 30
cook-brewing pot 77
Copper 15
Corinthians 11
cow milk 29
Cranberry juice 35
created 3
*cryptosporidium* 14
cryptoxanthine 36, 50
curry in soup 62

## D
Daniel 3
dehydration 8, 11
diabetes prevent 11, 20, 37, 76
dietary intake 3
digested food 10
digestive tract 9
diseases of sin 7
drinking water 7
DIY plumber 12, 13
DNA 46
Dark chocolate 56
Detoxification 65
Drugs-free 84

## E
Earth 9, Ecoli 13
Elijah 8
eternal life 18
Eve.improvemnt,3, 18, 35, 37
everlasting life 7

## F
faith 7, 8
Fibre.dietary;28,32, 34, 36, 37, 43, 46, 47
Fat 32, 34, 36, 37, 43, 45, 52, 67, 69
Fatigue 49
FIFMI church 3, 91
Filtered10
filtration cartridge 12
filtration systems 12
flavonoids 32, 33, 41
foetal.development 45
folic.acid.19.38,.45 71
Formic acid 32
footballers 22
fruits & juices 3, 83
fruit juice making machine 27, 54, 55

# INDEX

## G
gallate 20
Garden of Eden 18
Genesis 8, 9, 16, 32, 35, 60
glucobrassin 65
gluconasturtin 65
Gluconic acid 32
glucoraphane 65
Glucose oxidase 32
God 8, 53, 54, 84, 88
God's rain 8
Goitre 19
grace of God 3
green tea 20
grinding mill 74
gym exercises 22

## H
Hacha fruit 74
Hacha leaves 74
Hagar 9, 17
Happiness &wellbeing 44
health benefits 9, 18, 46
healthy drink 3, 7
healthy life style 8, 9, 25, 26, 27
healthy water 9
healthy.power.drinks 22
Herbicides 13
High.density .lipoprotein 36, 37, 67, 91
histamine 49
Holy spirit 7, 8, 18
Holy Trinity 94
Honey 29, 33, 80
Hops 75
Hot beverages 56
hot soup drinks 62
humble man of God 3
hydrogen peroxide 33
hydroxybenzoic.acid 40, 76
hydroxycinnamic acid 40, 76

## I
Immune.system.33,40, 46
Industrial centrifuge 30
Industrial system 15
inner soul 7
intestinal bacteria 19
invertase 32
iodine 19
Isaac 9
Ishmael 9

## J
Jacob's well 9
James 3, 8
JEHOVAH 7, 95
Jesus Christ 7, 20, 27, 84, 87, 88
John 7, 18
Joshua 32

## K
kidney 11
kidney filtration 10
Kings 8
Koro drinks

## L
Lactic acid 32, 78
lactobacter culture 76
Lactose-free.yogurt 80
Lead 15
LDL, 68, 92
lemon 72
lemon juice 48, 52
Lipo oxygenase 31
Lives 3
Lord Jesus Christ 8, 9
low calories 48
Low.density lipoprotein 36, 37
Luke 7, 8
lung cancer
Lutein 38, 50
lycopene 37, 38, 65

## M
magnesium 15, 19
Making yogurt 81
Malachi 95
malic acid 32
malnutrition 8
man's fertility 35
man's libido & vitality 34, 61
mango juice 43
manufacturing process 31
masvusvu 74, 75
Matthew 3
Melon juice 43
metabolic activity 19
Methodist Church 91
microfiltration 12
milk 17
millet 69, 73, 74
minerals 10, 36, 38, 52, 53
mixed fruits juice 43
modern science 7
monounsaturate FA 28
mulberries 69,
mushroom soup 62, 63
muzhanje (mazhanje)

## N
Naringen 48
Naringon 4
natural clean water 8
natural springs 9
New biotech. 77
niacin 36, 39
Noah 8, 37
Numbers 32, 33
Nutrients 3

## O
oesophagus cancer 20
oestrogen 30
Omega.3 (& Omega.6) FA 39, 40, 68
only begotten Son 7
Orange 43, 47, 48
organ cancers 17
osteoporosis 30
Other churches 91
our living God 7
our Saviour 9
Oxalates 36
oxidant properties 17
oxidation 17

## P
Pancreatic cancer 20
Panthocyanins 34
pantothenic acid 19
Peach juice 43, 52
peptides 10
pesticides 12
Phenols (poly) 13, 34, 40, 56, 7
physical exercises 89
physical health 7
Physiological & biochemical benefits 90
physiological benefits 3, 51, 52
phytoantioxidants 28, 30, 38, 41, 70

# INDEX

## P
phytochemicals 48, 50
Phytosterols 68
Pineapple 49
pineapple.juice 43, 52
pollutants –free 12
Polyhydroxylated FA 68
polyunsaturates 28
Pomegranate juice 34, 35, 43, 51, 52
Pomegranate peel 35,
Powering forward 87
Praying & fasting 89
Press ups 92
Preventing cancer, bps, obesity, diabetes 91
proanthocyanidins 37
probiotic supplements 19
Procyanidins 56
promised land 53
prostate cancer 17, 20, 28, 30, 34
protein 10, 28 ,32, 34, 35, 37, 43, 47, 51, 52, 56
protozoa 15
Proverbs 33
Prunes (plums dried) 43
Psalm 99
Pulicalagia polypeptide 51
purification 12
purified water 11
pyroglutamic acid 32

## R
rain water 9
Rebecca 9
Red guava 38
redeemed 7
rehydrate 11
rehydrating agent 12
rehydration 11, 64
rejuvenated 7, 16
remission of sins 7, 9
retinol 19
Rioflavin 36, 39
Romans 3

## S
Salicylic acid 36, 40
salts 10, 32, 34 35 ,36
Samaria woman 9
Sarah 16
Sarah 77
Saturated fats 28
Selenium 19
serotonin 44
Silver 15
smoke-free 84
sodium 15, 28, 35, 37, 43
sodium bicarbonate 31
Song of Solomon 54, 62
Sorghum 73, 74, 75
Soups 62, 63
soya beans 30
soya milk 29, 30
Speed training 86, 87
spiritual exercise 90
spiritual health 7
Spring water 8
sprinting practice 86
squash 92
Starter.cultures.,79, 80
Succinic.acid.32
Strawberries.40
Stilbenes 41
sugars 10, 28, 32, 34, 35, 36, 43, 47, 50, 52, 67, 69
superoxide dismutase 49

## T
table tennis 92
Talents 3
techniques of exercise 3
testosterone level 30
the Cross 7
theannine 20
thermometer 82, 83
Thomas 7
tissue poisoning 11
tithing.(tithe)90,91,95
to prosper 8
tomato 36, 37, 51, 52
tomato soup 66, 67
Total gallagyl 34
Total.ellagic.acids 34
Total.hydrolsable tannins 34, 35
toxic drugs 8
toxins 10, 11
tranquilizer 20
tribute 3
*tsime ra* Jacob

## U
unhealthy drinks 8
unsaturated.fatty acids 29
urinary tract 36

## V
vineyard 38
Vitamin A 18, 38, 39, 45, 46, 47, 49, 50, 63, 66, 68
Vitamin B1 18, 47, 48, 63
Vitamin B2 18
Vitamin B5 48
Vitamin B6 18, 39, 45, 49, 52, 69
Vitamin C 17, 18, 34, 36, 38, 39, 43, 45, 46, 47, 48, 49, 50, 51, 52, 64, 66, 67, 70
Vitamin D 18, 28
Vitamin E 36, 38, 45, 47, 51, 52
Vitamin K 39, 45, 51, 52, 65, 67, 70
Vitamin supplements 16
Vitamin.B12 18, 28,39,45, 52
Vitamins 10, 43, 51
Volatile acids 36
volatile organic C 13

## W
walk from sins 7
walk.run uphill 91
water filtration 12
water treatment 12
weight loss 28
weights lifting 93
world class athlete 84
world record 24

## X
Xanthins 51,53, 77

## Y
Yogurt 80, 81, 82, 83

## Z
Zea xanthin 51, 53, 71

# KEY STUDY NOTES FOR THE READER OF THE BOOK